Thyroid Cancer

About the NCCN Guidelines for Patients®

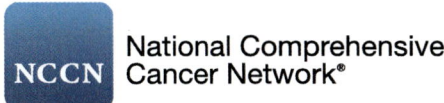

Did you know that top cancer centers across the United States work together to improve cancer care? This alliance of leading cancer centers is called the National Comprehensive Cancer Network® (NCCN®).

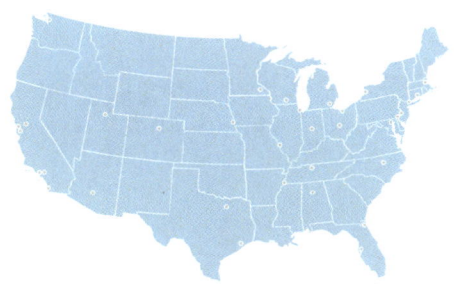

Cancer care is always changing. NCCN develops evidence-based cancer care recommendations used by health care providers worldwide. These frequently updated recommendations are the NCCN Clinical Practice Guidelines in Oncology (NCCN Guidelines®). The NCCN Guidelines for Patients plainly explain these expert recommendations for people with cancer and caregivers.

These NCCN Guidelines for Patients are based on the NCCN Clinical Practice Guidelines in Oncology (NCCN Guidelines®) for Thyroid Carcinoma, Version 3.2024 — June 18, 2024.

View the NCCN Guidelines for Patients free online
NCCN.org/patientguidelines

Find an NCCN Cancer Center near you
NCCN.org/cancercenters

Connect with us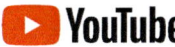

Supporters

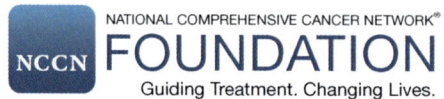

NCCN Guidelines for Patients are supported by funding from the NCCN Foundation®

NCCN Foundation gratefully acknowledges the following corporate supporters for helping to make available these NCCN Guidelines for Patients: Eisai Inc.; and Exelixis, Inc.

NCCN independently adapts, updates, and hosts the NCCN Guidelines for Patients. Our corporate supporters do not participate in the development of the NCCN Guidelines for Patients and are not responsible for the content and recommendations contained therein.

To make a gift or learn more, visit online or email

NCCNFoundation.org/donate   PatientGuidelines@NCCN.org

Contents

4 About thyroid cancer

8 Testing

12 Treatments

22 Papillary, follicular, and oncocytic carcinoma

33 Medullary thyroid cancer

41 Anaplastic thyroid cancer

51 Survivorship

55 Making treatment decisions

64 Words to know

66 NCCN Contributors

67 NCCN Cancer Centers

70 Index

© 2024 National Comprehensive Cancer Network, Inc. All rights reserved. NCCN Guidelines for Patients and illustrations herein may not be reproduced in any form for any purpose without the express written permission of NCCN. No one, including doctors or patients, may use the NCCN Guidelines for Patients for any commercial purpose and may not claim, represent, or imply that the NCCN Guidelines for Patients that have been modified in any manner are derived from, based on, related to, or arise out of the NCCN Guidelines for Patients. The NCCN Guidelines are a work in progress that may be redefined as often as new significant data become available. NCCN makes no warranties of any kind whatsoever regarding its content, use, or application and disclaims any responsibility for its application or use in any way.

NCCN Foundation seeks to support the millions of patients and their families affected by a cancer diagnosis by funding and distributing NCCN Guidelines for Patients. NCCN Foundation is also committed to advancing cancer treatment by funding the nation's promising doctors at the center of innovation in cancer research. For more details and the full library of patient and caregiver resources, visit NCCN.org/patients.

National Comprehensive Cancer Network (NCCN) and NCCN Foundation
3025 Chemical Road, Suite 100, Plymouth Meeting, PA 19462 USA

1
About thyroid cancer

5   The thyroid

6   Who is at risk?

7   Key points

There are different types of thyroid cancer. Most are curable with the right treatment. When possible, surgery is recommended for most thyroid cancers.

The thyroid

The thyroid is a butterfly-shaped gland in the front of the neck. It has 2 lobes, a right and a left. A thin piece of tissue called the isthmus connects the lobes.

The thyroid makes hormones. These substances are essential for the body to function properly. They circulate in the blood and help regulate body temperature, blood pressure, heart rate, weight, and metabolism (how fast food becomes fuel for your body).

The two main hormones made by the thyroid are thyroxine (T4) and triiodothyronine (T3). Together, these are often referred to simply as "thyroid hormone." The thyroid uses a mineral from your diet called iodine to produce these hormones. Certain foods and iodized salt contain iodine.

There are four pea-sized glands on the back of the thyroid gland. These parathyroid glands control the amount of calcium in your bloodstream.

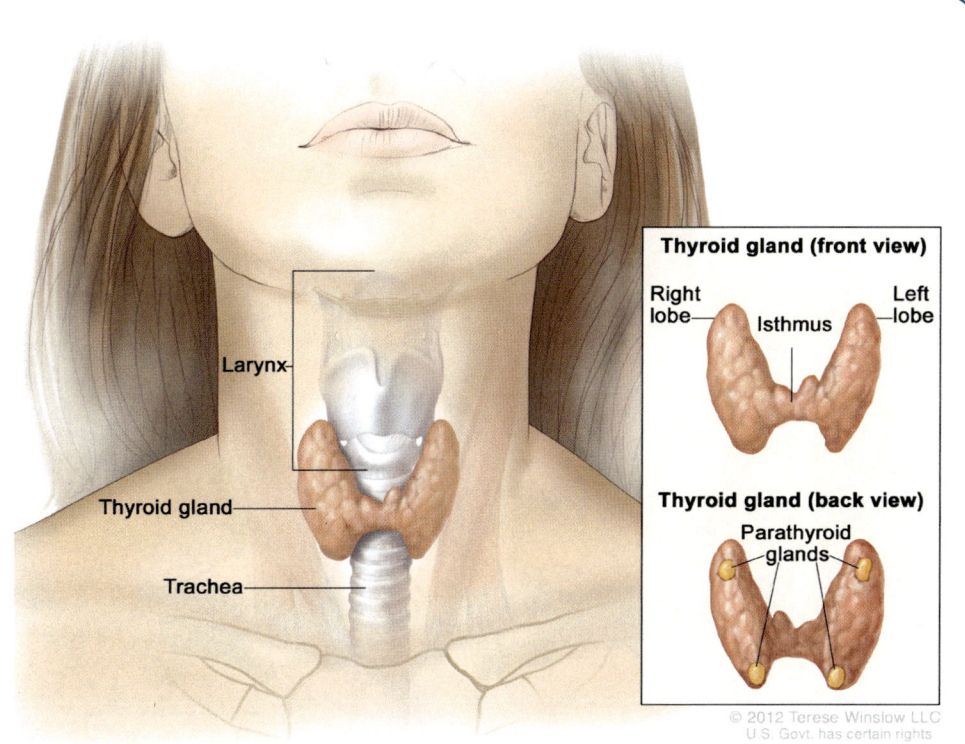

Thyroid gland

The thyroid is a butterfly-shaped gland in the lower front part of the neck. It makes hormones that control blood pressure, metabolism, and other body functions.

1 About thyroid cancer » Who is at risk?

Thyroid nodules

Thyroid nodules are small, often round areas of abnormal growth within the thyroid gland. Most are not cancerous. Very small nodules usually can't be seen or felt. Your provider may be able to see or feel a large nodule while examining your lower neck.

Most thyroid nodules don't cause symptoms. They are often found by imaging tests done for a different reason. Symptoms of a larger nodule could include:

- A visible lump in the neck
- Neck pain
- Voice changes
- Trouble breathing
- Problems swallowing

Who is at risk?

Those assigned female at birth are 3 times more likely to be diagnosed with a thyroid cancer compared to those assigned male at birth.

Compared to other cancers, thyroid cancer is often diagnosed earlier in adulthood. It is the most common cancer in adults aged 18 to 33 years. For more information on cancer in this group, see *NCCN Guidelines for Patients: Adolescent and Young Adult Cancer* at NCCN.org/patientguidelines and on the NCCN Patient Guides for Cancer app.

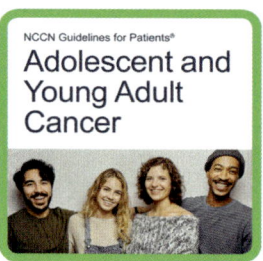

Anything that increases the chances of developing a disease is called a risk factor. The most well-known risk factors for thyroid cancer are described next. Most people with thyroid cancer have no known risk factors.

Radiation exposure

Anyone who has had radiation treatment to the head or neck in the past (to treat a childhood cancer, for example) is at increased risk of thyroid cancer.

Contact with large amounts of radiation in the environment as a result of a catastrophic event also increases the risk of developing a thyroid cancer.

1 About thyroid cancer » Key points

Family history

Most thyroid cancers are sporadic, meaning there is no clear cause or risk factor. Only a small number are hereditary, or the result of inherited gene mutations (changes).

A personal or family history of thyroid cancer or a related syndrome may increase the risk of thyroid cancer. Syndromes related to thyroid cancer include familial adenomatous polyposis (FAP), Carney complex, Cowden syndrome, and multiple endocrine neoplasia (MEN).

Cowden syndrome is also known as *PTEN* hamartoma tumor syndrome (PHTS). This inherited syndrome can cause follicular thyroid cancer, and other cancers and health problems. Tell your provider if you have a personal or family history of breast, endometrial, or colorectal cancer.

Key points

- The thyroid is a butterfly-shaped gland in the neck. It makes hormones that help regulate metabolism and other body functions.

- Thyroid cancers start as small, often round areas of abnormal growth called nodules. Most don't cause symptoms and are benign.

- Thyroid cancer is the most common cancer in adults aged 18 to 33 years. The most well-known risk factors are radiation exposure and a family history of thyroid cancer.

2
Testing

9 TSH test

9 Ultrasound

10 Biopsy

11 Key points

2 Testing » TSH test » Ultrasound

If a thyroid nodule is found or suspected, a thyroid-stimulating hormone (TSH) blood test and an ultrasound of the thyroid and neck are needed. Your doctor uses the results to decide whether a biopsy is needed.

TSH test

Thyroid stimulating hormone (TSH) is a hormone made by the pituitary gland, located near the base of the brain. TSH controls the hormones made by the thyroid.

A TSH blood test can't diagnose thyroid cancer. The level is checked to learn if the nodule is producing thyroid hormone. Nodules that make thyroid hormone are rarely cancerous.

A high TSH level usually means that the thyroid hormone levels are low.

A low TSH level usually means that the thyroid hormone levels are high. This is called hyperthyroidism or overactive thyroid. Your provider may order a radioactive iodine (RAI) uptake test.

Ultrasound

Ultrasound is the most common imaging technique used to look for thyroid cancer. It uses sound waves to form images showing the size, shape, and location of a thyroid nodule.

An ultrasound of the thyroid and neck is brief and painless. It is usually done lying down. A

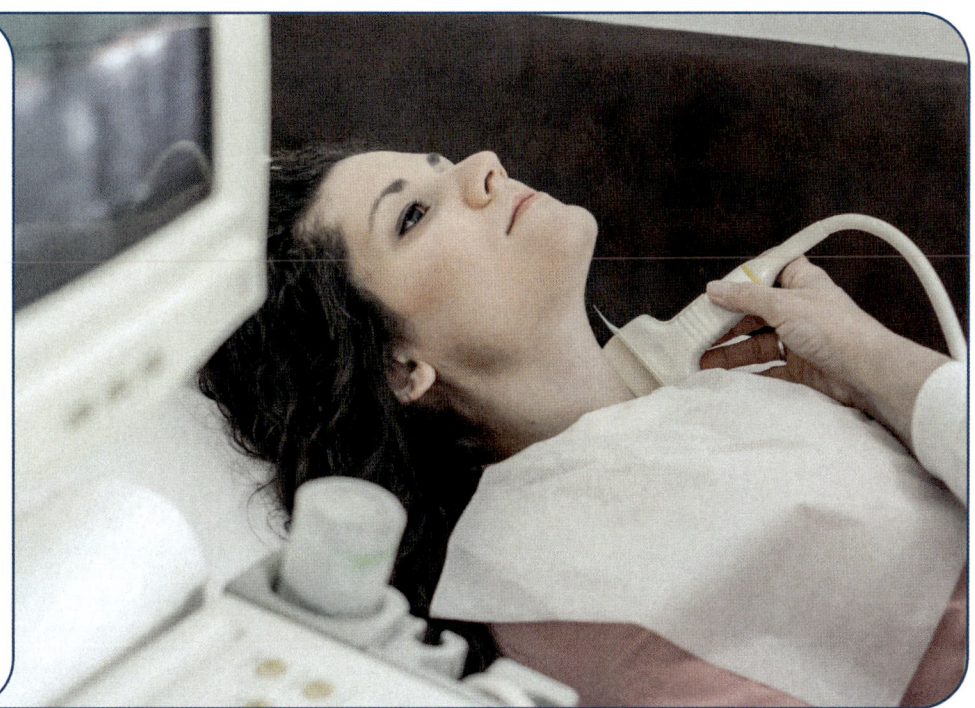

Ultrasound

An ultrasound of the thyroid and neck is one of the first tests ordered if a thyroid nodule is known or suspected.

hand-held device called an ultrasound probe is used. After a gel is applied to the skin, the probe is moved back and forth over the thyroid area.

If ultrasound finds any suspicious lymph nodes in the neck, further imaging with CT or MRI is recommended. A substance called contrast is used to make the pictures clearer.

Biopsy

A biopsy removes samples of fluid or tissue from the body to be tested. Your doctor will consider the nodule size and other features as seen on the ultrasound to determine if a biopsy is needed. Some nodules don't need to be biopsied and are monitored with ultrasound.

If a biopsy is needed, fine-needle aspiration (also called needle biopsy or FNA) is recommended. This method uses a thin needle to take small samples of suspicious thyroid nodules. Ultrasound is usually done at the same time to help pinpoint the suspicious areas.

Pathology review

The biopsy samples are sent to a pathologist. Pathologists are physicians with expertise in examining tissues and cells to diagnose disease. By examining the sample under a microscope, the pathologist is able to determine whether the nodule is cancerous, and if so, the cancer type.

In certain types of lesions, such as follicular and oncocytic tumors, fine-needle biopsy can identify the nature of the cells, but can't determine if the nodule is cancerous. For these lesions, surgery is often needed to make a final diagnosis. Now, molecular tests are available that can help determine whether the nodule is cancerous and whether surgery is necessary.

Papillary carcinoma is the most common type of thyroid cancer, followed by follicular carcinoma, then oncocytic. Papillary, follicular, and oncocytic carcinomas are known as the differentiated thyroid cancers. Differentiated cancers usually grow and spread slowly. Treatment of these types is addressed in Chapter 4.

Medullary thyroid cancer is the third most common type of thyroid cancer. This type can be inherited, meaning it can run in families. Medullary thyroid cancer is the focus of Chapter 5.

Anaplastic thyroid cancer is the most aggressive type of thyroid cancer. It is rare and most often affects older adults. This type is the focus of Chapter 6.

The type and other features of biopsied lesions are recorded in a pathology report. Ask for a copy of the report to have for your records. Your care team uses it to plan the next steps of care.

Key points

- Although most nodules aren't cancerous, a thyroid-stimulating hormone (TSH) test and ultrasound are recommended if a thyroid nodule is known or suspected.

- Your provider uses the ultrasound results to determine whether a needle biopsy is needed.

- Biopsy samples are sent to a pathologist. The pathologist determines whether the nodule is cancerous and, if so, the cancer type.

3
Treatments

13 Surgery

15 Radioactive iodine

16 Radiation therapy

18 Systemic therapy

19 Clinical trials

21 Key points

3 Treatments » Surgery

Surgery is the most common treatment for most thyroid cancers. However, active surveillance may be an option for some very-low-risk cancers. This involves closely monitoring the cancer instead of performing surgery right away.

Surgery

Surgery is the most effective treatment for thyroid cancer. Surgery may involve removing the entire thyroid gland, or just the half that contains cancer.

Lobectomy

A lobectomy removes the lobe of the thyroid that contains the cancerous nodule. The tissue connecting the two lobes (the isthmus) is also removed. While under general anesthesia, a small incision is made in the front of the neck to remove the cancerous lobe.

Lobectomy may be an option for some small and low-risk differentiated thyroid cancers.

Total thyroidectomy

A total thyroidectomy removes the entire thyroid gland. Lymph nodes near the thyroid are also removed if they are known or suspected to have cancer. This is called a neck dissection.

While under general anesthesia, a small incision is made in the front of the neck to remove the gland.

Most people stay in the hospital overnight after surgery. After being discharged, it is important to follow the instructions for at-home care. Contact your care team about any new or worsening side effects.

Long-term side effects of removing the thyroid can include:

› Low levels of calcium in the blood (hypoparathyroidism)

› Damage to the nerves that control your voice and swallowing

Thyroid hormone replacement therapy

After a total thyroidectomy, medicine is used to replace the hormones no longer being supplied by the thyroid. This is called thyroid hormone replacement therapy. It is needed lifelong in all people after total thyroidectomy. After a lobectomy, about 1 in 3 people need thyroid hormone therapy.

Levothyroxine (eg, Levoxyl; Synthroid) is the most commonly used thyroid hormone replacement therapy. The goal for most people is to keep the level of thyroid-stimulating hormone (TSH) in the low normal range.

For higher risk thyroid cancers, or if there are signs of recurrence, the TSH level is kept lower than the normal range (suppressed). This helps prevent thyroid cancer cells from growing or returning. Suppression is an important part of cancer therapy for most differentiated thyroid cancers.

3 Treatments » Surgery

Levothyroxine is taken as a pill once a day. It must be taken on an empty stomach, at least 30 mintutes prior to eating a meal. If not, it won't be adequately absorbed into the blood.

Finding the right dose can take some trial and error. If the dose isn't optimal, common side effects include:

- Anxiety
- Trouble sleeping
- Racing heart (with or without an abnormal heartbeat)
- Sweating

Blood tests are used to check the TSH level on a regular basis during thyroid replacement therapy. Your doctor can find the right dose of thyroid hormone for you by checking the TSH level and adjusting the dose as needed.

Too much levothyroxine can cause health problems, including:

- Weakened bones
- Heart rhythm problems
- Having too much thyroid hormone (thyrotoxicosis)

Calcium and vitamin D

Your provider may recommend taking calcium and vitamin D supplements to help strengthen your bones.

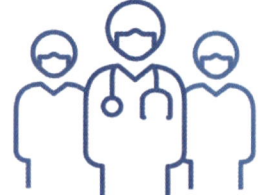

Treatment team

Treating thyroid cancer takes a team of experts. Your care team may include an endocrinologist, radiologist, nuclear medicine specialist, surgeon, radiation oncologist, and medical oncologist. You and your team will decide on a treatment plan that is best for you. This written course of action covers every phase of the treatment process.

3 Treatments » Radioactive iodine

Radioactive iodine

Radioactive iodine (RAI) therapy uses a form of radioactive iodine (iodine-131) to selectively kill thyroid cancer cells that take up ("eat") iodine.

The goal is to target only the thyroid cells in the neck (both cancer cells and any remaining normal thyroid cells) and elsewhere in the body while sparing healthy cells and tissues. RAI therapy may be used in the following situations:

- To lower the chances that a high-risk cancer returns after treatment
- To treat thyroid cancer that has spread within the body
- Shortly after thyroidectomy for some lower-risk cancers, using lower-dose iodine-131 (also known as remnant ablation)

RAI therapy is used after total thyroidectomy for differentiated thyroid cancers that take up iodine. It is generally only recommended for cancers at higher risk of coming back. RAI isn't effective against medullary or anaplastic thyroid cancer.

How is it given?

RAI therapy comes in liquid or pill form and is taken by mouth. You may be asked to eat a diet low in iodine for 1 to 2 weeks before starting this treatment.

You need a high level of TSH for RAI therapy. Thyroid hormone replacement may be stopped for a few weeks beforehand. If this isn't recommended for you, hormone injections of thyrotropin alfa (Thyrogen) can be used to increase the TSH level. Thyrogen activates iodine uptake so that hormone replacement can be continued therapy and imaging.

Possible side effects of RAI therapy include:

- Neck pain or swelling in glands near the jaw
- Nausea and vomiting
- Dry mouth or eyes
- Watery eyes
- Change in taste or smell

The dose of RAI therapy is often adjusted for children with thyroid cancer and people on dialysis for kidney disease. If any cancer can be removed by surgery, this will be considered before starting RAI therapy.

Safety measures

The radiation will exit your body through urine and other body fluids. This means that your body will give off small amounts of radiation after treatment. For a short time, you will need to take safety measures around others, especially children and pregnant people.

Whole-body RAI scan

After RAI, a whole-body radioiodine scan is performed to look for remaining thyroid tissue and "hidden" areas of thyroid cancer in the body. At some treatment centers, a whole-body scan is also done before RAI therapy. This imaging can be done using small doses of iodine-131 or a similar form of radioactive iodine called iodine-123.

Radiation therapy

Radiation therapy uses high-energy x-rays or particles to destroy small areas of cancer. To treat thyroid cancer, radiation is given using a large machine outside the body. This is called external beam radiation therapy (EBRT).

Radiation therapy is rarely used for papillary and follicular cancers. Anaplastic thyroid cancer, in contrast, is almost always treated with radiation therapy.

Radiation therapy may be used for thyroid cancer that can't be removed with surgery and doesn't respond to RAI therapy.

Radiation therapy can also relieve symptoms caused by cancer spread, such as difficulty or pain swallowing, loss of your voice, or pain or stiffness in your neck. It may also be helpful if the cancer has spread to another organ, such as the bones or brain, to stop the cancer from growing in that specific area.

You will first have a planning session called a simulation. You will be placed in the treatment position and a CT scan or other type of scan will be done. The images will be used to make a radiation plan tailored to your body and cancer.

During radiation treatment, you will lie on a table in the same position as during simulation. A technician will operate the machine from a nearby room, but will be able to see, hear, and speak with you at all times. You won't feel anything while the radiation is being delivered. One treatment session can take 30 to 60

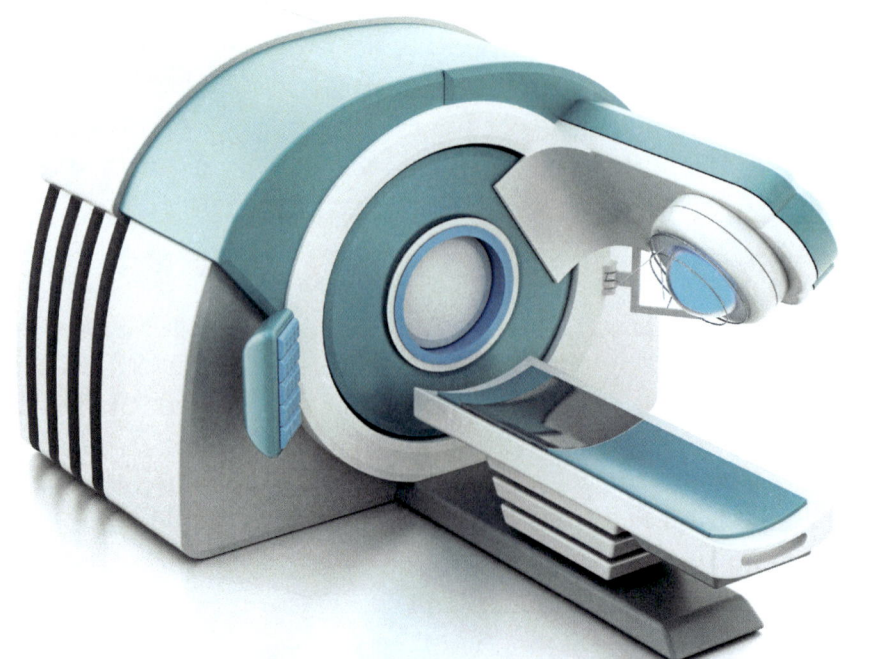

Radiation therapy

Radiation therapy uses high-energy radiation from x-rays, gamma rays, protons, and other sources to kill cancer cells and shrink tumors. It is also used to treat pain caused by the cancer.

minutes. It's common to have 5 sessions per week.

Common side effects of radiation to the neck area include:

- Skin rash or redness
- Problems swallowing
- Dry mouth
- Thick saliva
- Changes in taste
- Tiredness

While most side effects of radiation therapy start during treatment and stop shortly after it is over, some can occur years later. If your doctor recommends external radiation, they will discuss what to expect from treatment, including possible short- and long-term side effects.

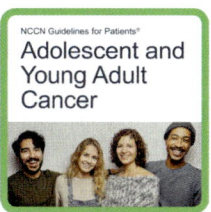

Fertility and family planning

If you want the option of having children after treatment or are unsure, tell your care team. Your doctor will discuss any fertility-related risks of your treatment plan with you. You may be referred for counseling about your fertility preservation options.

For more information on fertility and family planning, see the *NCCN Guidelines for Patients: Adolescent and Young Adult Cancer* at NCCN.org/patientguidelines and on the NCCN Patient Guides for Cancer app.

3 Treatments » Systemic therapy

Systemic therapy

Systemic therapy is treatment with substances that travel in the bloodstream, reaching and affecting cells throughout the body.

Chemotherapy, targeted therapy, and immunotherapy are types of systemic therapy.

Targeted therapy

Targeted therapies can target and attack specific types of cancer cells. They are generally only used for thyroid cancers that:

- Can't be treated with surgery or RAI therapy
- Have returned after treatment
- Have spread to areas far from the neck (metastasized) and are continuing to grow

The targeted therapies currently used for thyroid cancer are called kinase inhibitors. Most are capsules that you swallow.

Chemotherapy

Chemotherapy doesn't work well against most thyroid cancers. It may be used for cancer that isn't responding to other treatment, or that has spread to distant areas of the body. It is most often used in combination with radiation therapy for anaplastic thyroid cancer—the least common and most aggressive type.

Most chemotherapy medicines are put directly into the bloodstream through a vein.

Systemic therapy side effects

Side effects of systemic therapy can include:

- Tiredness (fatigue)
- Nausea and vomiting
- Diarrhea
- Constipation
- Hair loss
- Mouth sores
- Loss of appetite
- Low blood cell counts (white cells, red cells, and platelets)

Side effects seen more often with targeted therapy include body aches, rash, high blood pressure, and abnormal bleeding.

Some targeted therapies have serious side effects that can affect your heart, skin, and digestive system. If systemic therapy is planned, ask your care team for a complete list of potential side effects.

Most side effects only occur during cancer treatment. But, some can start years later. For example, long-term side effects of chemotherapy can include other cancers, heart disease, and not being able to have children.

3 Treatments » Clinical trials

Clinical trials

A clinical trial is a type of medical research study. After being developed and tested in a laboratory, potential new ways of fighting cancer need to be studied in people. If found to be safe and effective in a clinical trial, a drug, device, or treatment approach may be approved by the U.S. FDA.

Everyone with cancer should carefully consider all of the treatment options available for their cancer type, including standard treatments and clinical trials. Talk to your doctor about whether a clinical trial may make sense for you.

Phases

Most cancer clinical trials focus on treatment. Treatment trials are done in phases.

- **Phase 1** trials study the safety and side effects of an investigational drug or treatment approach.
- **Phase 2** trials study how well the drug or approach works against a specific type of cancer.
- **Phase 3** trials test the drug or approach against a standard treatment. If the results are good, it may be approved by the FDA.
- **Phase 4** trials study the long-term safety and benefit of an FDA-approved treatment.

Who can enroll?

Every clinical trial has rules for joining, called eligibility criteria. The rules may be about age, cancer type and stage, treatment history, or general health. These requirements ensure that participants are alike in specific ways and that the trial is as safe as possible for the participants.

Informed consent

Clinical trials are managed by a group of experts called a research team. The research team will review the study with you in detail, including its purpose and the risks and benefits of joining. All of this information is also provided in an informed consent form. Read the form carefully and ask questions before signing it. Take time to discuss with family, friends, or others you trust. Keep in mind that you can leave and seek treatment outside of the clinical trial at any time.

Start the conversation

Don't wait for your doctor to bring up clinical trials. Start the conversation and learn about all of your treatment options. If you find a study that you may be eligible for, ask your treatment team if you meet the requirements. Try not to be discouraged if you cannot join. New clinical trials are always becoming available.

Frequently asked questions

There are many myths and misconceptions surrounding clinical trials. The possible benefits and risks are not well understood by many people with cancer.

Will I get a placebo?
Placebos (inactive versions of real medicines) are almost never used alone in cancer clinical trials. It is common to receive either a placebo with a standard treatment, or a new drug with a standard treatment. You will be informed,

3 Treatments » Clinical trials

verbally and in writing, if a placebo is part of a clinical trial before you enroll.

Are clinical trials free?

There is no fee to enroll in a clinical trial. The study sponsor pays for research-related costs, including the study drug. You may, however, have costs indirectly related to the trial, such as the cost of transportation or childcare due to extra appointments. During the trial, you will continue to receive standard cancer care. This care is billed to—and often covered by—insurance. You are responsible for copays and any costs for this care that are not covered by your insurance.

Finding a clinical trial

In the United States

NCCN Cancer Centers
NCCN.org/cancercenters

The National Cancer Institute (NCI)
cancer.gov/about-cancer/treatment/clinical-trials/search

Worldwide

The U.S. National Library of Medicine (NLM)
clinicaltrials.gov

Need help finding a clinical trial?

NCI's Cancer Information Service (CIS)
1.800.4.CANCER (1.800.422.6237)
cancer.gov/contact

Key points

- Your treatment team may include an endocrinologist, radiologist, nuclear medicine doctor, surgeon, radiation oncologist, and medical oncologist.

- Surgery is the main treatment for thyroid cancer. Active surveillance may be an option for very-low-risk cancers. RAI therapy may be used after total thyroidectomy to kill any remaining cancer cells.

- Thyroid hormone replacement therapy with levothyroxine is needed lifelong after total thyroidectomy. About 1 in 3 people need hormone replacement after a lobectomy.

- External beam radiation therapy (EBRT) is used for more aggressive (anaplastic), recurrent, or metastatic cancers that can't be removed surgically.

- Targeted therapy may be an option for thyroid cancers that don't respond to other treatments, or that have metastasized and are continuing to grow.

- Clinical trials provide access to investigational treatments that may, in time, be approved by the U.S. FDA.

4 Papillary, follicular, and oncocytic carcinoma

23 Papillary thyroid cancer

26 Follicular and oncocytic carcinoma

27 Radioactive iodine therapy

28 Monitoring and follow-up care

30 Recurrence

31 Metastatic cancer

32 Key points

4 Papillary, follicular, and oncocytic carcinoma » Papillary thyroid cancer

Papillary, follicular, and oncocytic carcinoma are known as differentiated thyroid cancers. These cancers usually grow slowly and have good treatment outcomes.

Differentiated thyroid cancers are treated with surgery to remove all or part of the thyroid. For many years, total thyroidectomy was the standard treatment for all thyroid cancers. Today, it remains a treatment option for everyone with thyroid cancer.

However, newer research shows that lobectomy may be just as effective for treating small, low-risk cancers that haven't grown or spread beyond the thyroid. A potential benefit of lobectomy is that thyroid hormone replacement therapy may not be needed. Or, a lower dose may be needed.

Papillary thyroid cancer

Papillary thyroid carcinoma (PTC) is the most common of all the thyroid cancers. The most common subtype is "classic type." Other subtypes that may grow and spread more quickly include:

- Follicular variant of papillary thyroid cancer
- Tall-cell/columnar cell
- Hobnail
- Diffuse sclerosing

Is surgery always needed?

Some small papillary tumors (no bigger than a pea) may be safely monitored without surgery. This approach is known as active surveillance. The size of the cancer is monitored using ultrasound.

For active surveillance to be an option, there also can't be any nearby lymph nodes suspicious for cancer, and the tumor can't be in a high-risk location (such as the back of the thyroid, butting up against the trachea).

Thyroidectomy or lobectomy?

If surgery is needed, either a total thyroidectomy or lobectomy is performed.

Some papillary cancers should always be treated with total thyroidectomy. A total thyroidectomy is recommended for papillary cancers that have grown or spread beyond the thyroid—whether into the neck, to nearby lymph nodes, or to distant areas.

4 Papillary, follicular, and oncocytic carcinoma » Papillary thyroid cancer

Tumors larger than 4 centimeters (cm) (about the size of a walnut) and high-risk types of papillary cancer should also be treated with total thyroidectomy. Lymph nodes near the thyroid that are known to have cancer are also removed during surgery.

There are other reasons your doctor may recommend a total thyroidectomy. Factors such as whether the neck area was ever treated with radiation therapy will be considered.

If the cancer is small and noninvasive, lobectomy may be a treatment option in addition to thyroidectomy. Treatment with lobectomy is preferred if the following criteria are met:

- You've never had radiation therapy
- The cancer hasn't spread at all beyond the thyroid.
- The tumor is 1 to 4 cm in size.

The extent of the cancer can't be fully known until the surgeon sees the thyroid, tumor, and surrounding areas first-hand, as well as the results of the pathologic exam of the removed tissues. If the cancer is larger or more invasive than expected during a lobectomy, the decision is usually made during surgery to remove the entire thyroid.

After total thyroidectomy

If the results of surgery are very good, radioactive iodine (RAI) therapy is sometimes used to kill cancer cells left in the body.

If a concerning amount of cancer remains after surgery, treatment options may include:

- Another surgery
- RAI therapy
- Radiation therapy
- Systemic therapy
- Monitoring

After treatment with 1 or more of the above, thyroid hormone replacement therapy with levothyroxine is started. This keeps the thyroid-stimulating hormone (TSH) level low or normal.

After lobectomy

After a lobectomy, everything that was removed or sampled (biopsied) during surgery is examined and tested. If examination of the tumor, other tissue, or lymph nodes by a pathologist finds certain concerning or high-risk features, another surgery to remove the rest of the thyroid (completion thyroidectomy) is recommended.

If the results of surgery and pathologic examination are very good and no high-risk features are found, more surgery isn't usually needed. Your doctor may recommend thyroid hormone replacement therapy with levothyroxine to keep the TSH level low or normal. This is on a case-by-case basis.

Because the thyroid continues to make hormones after a lobectomy, hormone replacement therapy isn't always needed.

NIFTP

Pathologic examination after surgery may find that the tumor is a noninvasive follicular thyroid neoplasm with papillary-like nuclear features (NIFTP). A NIFTP is a low-risk, noninvasive thyroid tumor.

NIFTP was previously known as the encapsulated follicular variant of papillary thyroid cancer. No further treatment is needed after an NIFTP is surgically removed.

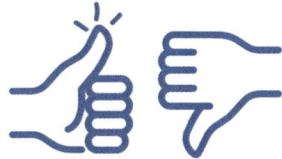

Let us know what you think!

Please take a moment to complete an online survey about the NCCN Guidelines for Patients.

NCCN.org/patients/response

4 Papillary, follicular, and oncocytic carcinoma » Follicular and oncocytic carcinoma

Follicular and oncocytic carcinoma

Follicular thyroid carcinoma (FTC) is the second most common type of thyroid cancer.

Oncocytic carcinoma is uncommon. This type was formerly known as Hürthle cell carcinoma (HCC). Compared to papillary and follicular tumors, oncocytic carcinoma is more likely to spread to lymph nodes by the time it is found.

Both follicular and oncocytic thyroid cancers are known for invading blood vessels in and around the thyroid. These cancers can't be diagnosed with a needle biopsy alone. Fine-needle aspiration (FNA) can only suggest these types.

In order to be diagnosed as follicular or oncocytic cancer, the cancer must have grown into veins or arteries in and around the thyroid, or into the outer layer of the tumor. This can be learned by pathologic examination of the removed thyroid, or in some cases with genetic testing of the biopsy sample.

Total thyroidectomy or lobectomy?

A total thyroidectomy is recommended for a suspected follicular or oncocytic tumor that has grown beyond the thyroid. The surgeon will also remove any nearby lymph nodes known to have cancer. Your provider may also recommend total thyroidectomy if the tumor is larger than 4 cm.

If the cancer hasn't spread beyond the thyroid, lobectomy may be a treatment option in addition to thyroidectomy. The extent of the cancer can't be fully known until the surgeon sees the thyroid, tumor, and surrounding areas first-hand, as well as the results of the pathologic examination of the removed tissues.

If the cancer is more invasive than expected during a lobectomy, the decision is usually made during surgery to remove the entire thyroid.

After total thyroidectomy

After surgery, everything that was removed or sampled (biopsied) is examined by a pathologist. Pathologic examination may find that the tumor is benign (not cancer). In this case, no more cancer treatment is needed. Lifelong thyroid hormone replacement therapy is needed, however.

If pathologic examination confirms follicular or oncocytic thyroid cancer, further treatment depends on the results of surgery. RAI therapy may be used to kill cancer cells left in the body. See the next page for more information.

If a concerning amount of cancer remains after surgery, there is more than one possibility. Options may include:

- Another surgery (preferred, if possible)
- RAI therapy
- Radiation therapy
- Systemic therapy
- Monitoring

After treatment with one or more of the above, hormone replacement therapy with levothyroxine is started. Hormone replacement therapy keeps the TSH level low or normal.

4 Papillary, follicular, and oncocytic carcinoma » Radioactive iodine therapy

After lobectomy

Depending on the extent of cancer observed during surgery and the results of pathologic examination, you may have more surgery to remove the rest of the thyroid. If the cancer is invasive, removing the rest of the thyroid is recommended.

For less invasive or minimally invasive cancer, surgery to remove the rest of the thyroid is one option. An alternative is to take a watch-and-wait approach and monitor the cancer. If this option is planned, you may receive levothyroxine to keep your TSH level low or normal. This is on a case-by-case basis. Because the thyroid continues to make hormones after a lobectomy, hormone replacement therapy isn't always needed.

If the nodule removed during lobectomy is benign, monitoring is recommended. In some cases, you may receive levothyroxine to keep your TSH level normal.

Radioactive iodine therapy

If all or most of the cancer was removed during total thyroidectomy, RAI therapy may be an option to kill thyroid cancer cells left in the body.

Your provider will consider the following factors to help decide if RAI may be helpful:

› The size of the tumor
› The tumor subtype
› Whether the cancer invaded lymph or blood vessels
› Whether the cancer has spread to lymph nodes
› The thyroglobulin (Tg) level after surgery
› Age at diagnosis

RAI therapy is usually recommended if **any** of the following is true:

› The cancer had spread significantly beyond the thyroid
› The cancer had invaded blood vessels (applies to follicular and oncocytic tumors)
› The Tg level was high 6 to 12 weeks after surgery
› There were large, or more than 5, lymph nodes with cancer
› The tumor is a differentiated high-grade carcinoma

Monitoring and follow-up care

Follow-up testing and surveillance are somewhat different after lobectomy versus after total thyroidectomy.

After total thyroidectomy

Short-term follow-up after total thyroidectomy involves a physical exam and blood tests. A neck ultrasound is also recommended 6 to 12 months after surgery. More information on blood tests is provided on the next page.

If you had RAI therapy after total thyroidectomy, you may have whole-body RAI imaging to look for cancer after treatment. It may be helpful for high-risk patients, those with metastases that took up iodine, or those with abnormal blood or ultrasound results.

Blood tests

Blood testing will measure the levels of the following:

- Thyroid-stimulating hormone (TSH)
- Thyroglobulin (Tg)
- Anti-thyroglobulin antibodies (Tg ab)

Thyroglobulin (Tg) is only made by thyroid tissue. If the thyroid is removed, there shouldn't be any Tg in the blood. Therefore, checking the Tg level can serve as a way to monitor for the return of cancer. If the Tg level rises, it could be a sign that further testing is needed to check for recurrence.

A small number of people with thyroid cancer make antibodies in response to Tg. These anti-Tg antibodies in blood can interfere with the Tg level. If the anti-Tg antibody level goes down, it may be a sign that treatment is working. If

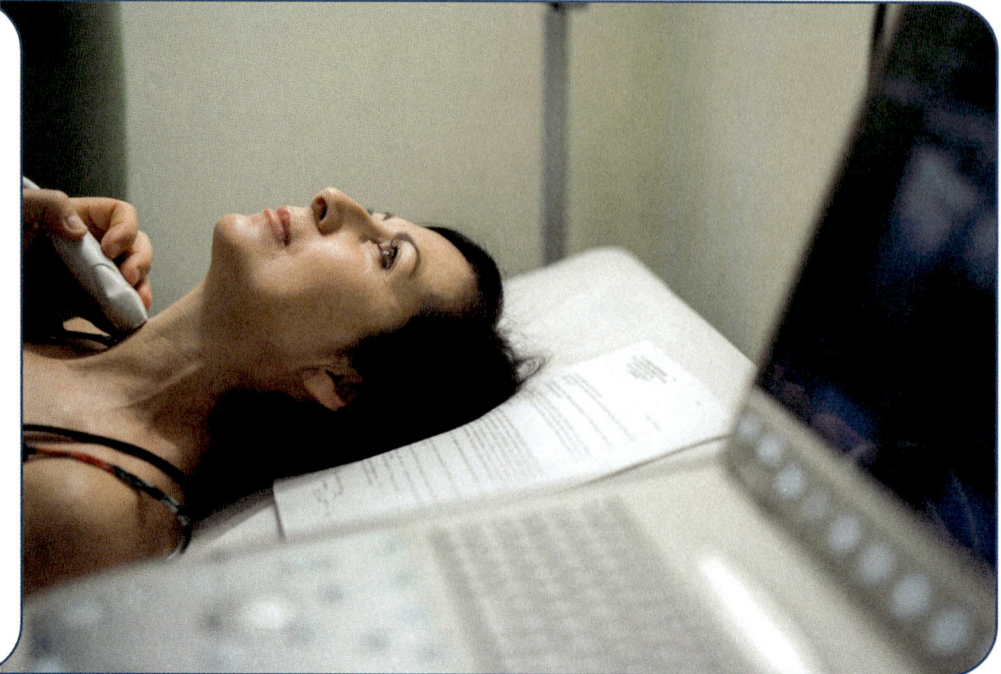

Neck ultrasound

Neck ultrasound is used to monitor for the return of thyroid cancer. Talk to your care team about how often you need to have ultrasounds.

4 Papillary, follicular, and oncocytic carcinoma » Monitoring and follow-up care

it goes up, further testing should be done to check for cancer recurrence.

Long-term monitoring

If follow-up test results are normal, it is considered no evidence of disease (NED). In those with NED, longer-term surveillance includes physical exams, blood tests (TSH, Tg, and Tg ab), and periodic neck ultrasound.

If there is reason to suspect the cancer has returned, you may have additional lab work, additional neck ultrasounds, TSH-stimulated testing (testing while thyroid hormone is stopped), or imaging procedures such as CT or MRI.

After lobectomy

Short-term follow-up after lobectomy involves a physical exam and TSH blood test. A neck ultrasound is also recommended 6 to 12 months after surgery. Unlike after total thyroidectomy, Tg testing isn't helpful after lobectomy.

If there is no evidence of disease, longer-term surveillance includes physical exams, TSH blood tests, and neck ultrasound. Talk to your care team about how often you need to have ultrasounds.

Survivorship

In addition to surveillance testing, a range of other care is important for cancer survivors. See *Chapter 7: Survivorship* for more information.

Recurrence

Although the thyroid has been removed, cancer can return to the neck or to areas far from the neck. The return of cancer after treatment is called recurrence.

Biomarker testing

Biomarkers are targetable features of a cancer. Many are mutations (changes) in the DNA of the cancer cells. For thyroid cancers with 1 or more specific biomarkers, targeted therapy or immunotherapy may be a treatment option if needed.

Biomarker testing involves analyzing a piece of tumor tissue in a lab or testing a sample of blood. Testing for the following biomarkers is recommended for recurrent, advanced, or metastatic cancers that can't be treated with RAI therapy:

- *ALK* gene fusion
- *NTRK* gene fusion
- *BRAF* gene mutations
- *RET* gene fusion (found in some medullary thyroid cancers)
- Mismatch repair deficiency (dMMR)
- Microsatellite instability-high (MSI-H)
- Tumor mutational burden-high (TMB-H)

Your provider may test for these individually or as part of a group. Testing for many biomarkers at one time is called next-generation sequencing (NGS).

Cancer that returns to the neck

If the cancer can be removed based on its size and location, surgery is the preferred treatment. For cancers that take up iodine, treatment with RAI therapy will also be considered.

But, treatment isn't always needed. If the cancer isn't getting worse and isn't close to any critical structures, your provider may recommend close monitoring instead of treatment.

If the cancer can't be removed with surgery, doesn't take up iodine, and is getting worse (progressing), treatment with radiation therapy, targeted therapy, or both may be an option.

The preferred targeted therapy for cancer that can't be removed with surgery and is progressing is lenvatinib (Lenvima). Another recommended option is sorafenib (Nexavar). If the cancer gets worse after treatment with 1 or both of these, cabozantinib (Cabometyx) is recommended.

For cancers with certain gene mutations or other features, biomarker-based therapy may also be an option for recurrence. See **Guide 1** on the next page.

If the therapies discussed above aren't available or appropriate, joining a clinical trial is strongly encouraged.

Metastatic cancer

Thyroid cancer that spreads to areas far from the neck is known as metastatic. Metastatic tumors can form anywhere but are most common in the lungs, liver, muscles, bones, brain, and spinal cord.

If the cancer takes up iodine, RAI therapy is recommended to treat metastatic papillary, follicular, or oncocytic thyroid cancers. Local therapies, such as radiation therapy, may also be used to treat areas of cancer directly.

If RAI therapy isn't an option

If the cancer doesn't take up iodine, targeted therapy may be an option. But, if the metastatic tumors are growing slowly (or not at all) and aren't causing symptoms, monitoring the cancer may be a better option. Some people live with their thyroid cancer for months or years without needing treatment. You will continue to take levothyroxine to keep your TSH level down.

To learn whether you are eligible for treatment with a targeted therapy or immunotherapy, biomarker testing is recommended. This testing is described in more detail on page 30. Recommended targeted therapies for metastatic cancer that can't be treated with surgery or RAI are listed in **Guide 1**.

Other systemic therapies are available and may be recommended if those listed in Guide 1 aren't available or appropriate. Joining a clinical trial is strongly encouraged for everyone with metastatic thyroid cancer.

Guide 1
Biomarker-based treatment

Biomarker	Available therapies
BRAF V600E gene mutation	Dabrafenib (Tafinlar) and trametinib (Mekinist)
NTRK gene fusion	• Larotrectinib (Vitrakvi) • Entrectinib (Rozlytrek)
RET gene fusion	• Selpercatinib (Retevmo) • Pralsetinib (Gavreto)
TMB-H	Pembrolizumab (Keytruda)
dMMR/MSI-H	Pembrolizumab (Keytruda)

Local therapies

Small tumors can be treated directly using 1 or more types of local therapy. If the cancer has only spread to a limited number of sites, or has spread to bone and/or is causing symptoms, it may be possible to remove or destroy the metastases with surgery and/or radiation therapy.

Ablation is another method used to treat small bone tumors. In ethanol ablation, a concentrated alcohol solution is injected into the neck to kill cancer cells. Cryoablation involves applying an extremely cold wand directly into the tumor.

Radiofrequency ablation uses radiofrequency waves that generate heat to kill cancer cells. Stereotactic body radiation therapy (SBRT) is a special ablative radiation technique that delivers high doses of radiation to precise areas to kill cancer cells.

If the cancer has spread to your bones, your provider may recommend intravenous bisphosphonate or denosumab. These are bone-strengthening medications that can slow damage caused by bone tumors and help relieve symptoms.

If the cancer has spread to the brain or spinal cord, treatment options may include surgery to remove the metastases. Stereotactic radiosurgery (SRS) is a non-surgical and highly precise type of radiation therapy that can be used to treat small brain or spine tumors. Whole brain radiation therapy (WBRT) is another type of EBRT used to treat cancer in the brain in which radiation is given to the whole brain.

Supportive care

Supportive care is essential for people with metastatic thyroid cancer. In addition to providing relief from symptoms, supportive care can provide emotional, spiritual, and social support.

Key points

- Papillary, follicular, and oncocytic carcinoma are differentiated thyroid cancers. Differentiated cancers tend to grow and spread slowly. They usually have good treatment outcomes.

- Total thyroidectomy is an option for all of the differentiated cancers. Lobectomy may also be an option for small, low-risk cancers.

- Total thyroidectomy is recommended for any cancer that has grown or spread beyond the thyroid. RAI therapy may follow.

- After a total thyroidectomy, lifelong thyroid hormone replacement therapy is needed. Levothyroxine is almost always used.

- Hormone replacement therapy isn't always needed after lobectomy, because the remaining lobe of the thyroid is still making hormones.

- Recurrences are usually diagnosed by lab or imaging studies and treated with some combination of surgery, RAI, EBRT, or systemic therapy. Treatment is individualized.

5
Medullary thyroid cancer

34 Testing

35 Staging

36 Treatment

37 After surgery

38 If cancer returns to the neck

39 Metastatic cancer

40 Key points

The most common types of thyroid cancer start in follicular cells, where thyroid hormone is made. Medullary thyroid carcinoma (MTC) starts in C cells. C cells make a different hormone called calcitonin. MTC behaves somewhat differently than differentiated thyroid cancers.

About 1 in 4 medullary thyroid cancers is caused by a pathogenic variant (a change) in the RET gene. These changes are also called mutations.

RET mutations can be passed from parent to child (inherited). The hereditary form of medullary thyroid cancer is known as multiple endocrine neoplasia type 2 (MEN2).

Compared to sporadic (non-inherited) medullary thyroid cancer, the hereditary form tends to start at a much younger age and behave more aggressively. For this reason, the thyroid may be removed at a very young age in infants and children known to have a RET mutation.

Inherited medullary thyroid cancer also tends to spread to lymph nodes or distant parts of the body earlier and more often than non-hereditary medullary thyroid cancer. The cancer can spread to the lungs, liver, or bones.

There are different mutations of the RET gene. Some are more likely to cause thyroid cancer than others. Some are also associated with more aggressive thyroid cancer. The specific RET mutation can affect:

> The overall chance of developing thyroid cancer

> When thyroid cancer starts

> How aggressive/fast-growing the thyroid cancer will be

MEN2A, which includes familial medullary thyroid carcinoma (FMTC), is generally considered moderate risk. In people with MEN2A the parathyroid glands can make too many hormones and may need to be removed. MEN2B is caused by higher-risk mutations of the RET gene.

Those with hereditary medullary thyroid cancer are at risk for developing a type of adrenal cancer called pheochromocytoma.

Testing

If a needle biopsy (fine-needle aspiration or FNA) diagnoses medullary thyroid cancer, more testing will be ordered. Genetic testing and counseling, blood and lab tests, and imaging procedures are used to help plan treatment.

Genetic testing and counseling

Everyone with medullary thyroid cancer found by FNA should be tested for inherited (called germline) mutations of the RET gene. Those who have a RET mutation will be referred to a genetic counselor.

This specially trained health professional can explain the test results and provide information, counseling, and support. The counselor can explain what the results mean for members of your family, including whether they should seek testing for the same mutation.

Seeing a genetic counselor is also encouraged before having any testing performed. It can help prepare you for the possible outcomes and what they mean for you and your loved ones.

Blood tests

Before treatment, blood tests will be ordered to measure the levels of calcitonin, calcium, and carcinoembryonic antigen (CEA). CEA is a protein that can be found in the blood of people with medullary thyroid cancer and some other cancers. It may also be used to check treatment results and monitor for the return of cancer.

Imaging

If an ultrasound of the thyroid and neck hasn't yet been done, it is recommended before surgery. Some people will also have an exam of the voice box and vocal cords. This is called laryngoscopy. A vocal cord exam may be helpful in patients with voice changes, invasive cancer, or bulky (large) cancer in the middle of the neck. It may also be ordered in those who have had surgery involving nerves near the voice box.

Additional imaging is needed for metastatic cancer. This may include computed tomography (CT), magnetic resonance imaging (MRI), positron emission tomography (PET), bone scan, and whole-body MRI.

Staging

The results of the testing described above are used to determine the spread of cancer in the body, also known as the cancer stage. While the stage of medullary thyroid cancer provides helpful information about the extent and outlook of the cancer, it doesn't guide your treatment. This is because surgery is recommended for all MTCs.

In the early stages of medullary thyroid cancer, the tumor has not spread beyond the thyroid. A 2 cm or smaller tumor (about the size of a peanut) is stage 1.

In stage 2 MTC the tumor is larger than 2 cm. It may have grown into muscles next to the thyroid. In stage 3, cancer has spread to nearby lymph nodes. The tumor itself may be small or large.

There are 3 categories of stage 4 medullary thyroid cancer. Stage 4A is moderately advanced disease. The tumor has grown extensively into the neck, or has spread to lymph nodes far from the thyroid.

Stage 4B is considered very advanced disease. Although there is no cancer in nearby lymph nodes, the tumor has invaded critical areas or structures such as the spine, large blood vessels, or the carotid artery.

Stage 4C is the most advanced stage, metastatic. The cancer has spread to areas of the body far from the thyroid.

Treatment

Sporadic MTC

Sporadic (non-hereditary) medullary thyroid cancer is treated with surgery to remove the entire thyroid (total thyroidectomy). Depending on the size and location of the tumor, the surgeon may also remove nearby lymph nodes that are known or suspected to have cancer. This is known as neck dissection. Neck dissection may not be needed for some tumors smaller than 1 cm (about the size of a pea).

Levothyroxine is given after surgery to replace the hormones no longer being supplied by the thyroid. Hormone replacement therapy is generally needed lifelong after a thyroidectomy. See the next page for information on what to expect after surgery.

Hereditary MTC

Treatment of both forms of hereditary medullary thyroid cancer (MEN2A and MEN2B) is similar and is described next.

MEN2A

MEN2A, which includes familial thyroid cancer, is treated using total thyroidectomy. In infants or young children known to have this type of inherited medullary thyroid cancer, it is recommended that the thyroid be removed at an early age. The timing of surgery is based on the aggressiveness of the specific inherited *RET* mutation.

Lymph nodes near the thyroid may also be removed during surgery. Reasons for removing lymph nodes may include high calcitonin or CEA levels before surgery, or abnormal ultrasound results.

If the parathyroid glands are making too much parathyroid hormone, one or more of the glands may be removed during surgery. Some or all of the tissue of individual parathyroid glands may be removed.

Parathyroid tissue can be removed and transplanted into another area of the body, such as the forearm. Over time, the tissue begins to make hormones again. Parathyroid gland tissue can also be frozen and stored outside the body (cryopreservation). This preserves the tissue so that it can be put back into the body at a later date.

Levothyroxine is given after surgery to replace the hormones no longer being supplied by the thyroid. Hormone replacement therapy is generally needed lifelong after a thyroidectomy.

MEN2B

Like MEN2A, MEN2B is treated using total thyroidectomy. In infants known to have this type of inherited medullary thyroid cancer, it is recommended that the thyroid be removed by age 1.

In addition to the thyroid gland, any neck lymph nodes known or suspected to have cancer will be removed. Lymph nodes without cancer may also be removed in order to prevent cancer cells from spreading to them.

Levothyroxine is given after surgery to replace the hormones no longer being supplied by the thyroid. Hormone replacement therapy is generally needed lifelong after a thyroidectomy.

After surgery

After a thyroidectomy, the best way to monitor for the return of medullary thyroid cancer is to check the levels of calcitonin and CEA on a regular basis. The calcitonin level after surgery is particularly important. The lower the calcitonin level, the better.

The first blood test will take place 2 to 3 months after surgery. It is important to wait a few months before testing because it takes time for the calcitonin level to drop after the thyroid is removed.

Normal blood test results

If the first blood test after surgery does not detect calcitonin and CEA is within normal range, the cancer is likely cured. Going forward, the calcitonin and CEA levels should be measured every year. If either level begins to rise, further testing and workup are needed.

In addition to annual calcitonin and CEA testing, yearly testing for pheochromocytoma is recommended for people with an inherited medullary thyroid cancer (MEN2A or MEN2B). In those with MEN2A, yearly testing for hyperparathyroidism is also recommended.

Abnormal blood test results

If the first blood test after surgery finds calcitonin, or if the CEA level is high, the cancer may not have been completely removed during surgery. Or it may have returned or spread.

Your provider may order imaging tests of your neck, liver, chest, and/or bones. If imaging results show cancer, or if you are having symptoms, see the next page.

If the imaging tests don't find anything concerning and you aren't having symptoms, you will be closely monitored. Blood tests to measure calcitonin and CEA are recommended every 6 to 12 months. Depending on how quickly the levels are rising, imaging procedures or more frequent testing may be needed. Sometimes another surgery is considered to remove remaining cancer.

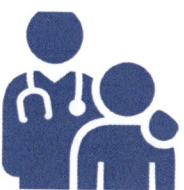

When surgery is planned in a child, thyroidectomy should be performed by a surgeon and a team experienced in performing pediatric thyroid surgery.

If cancer returns to the neck

If MTC returns to the neck area, biomarker (also called somatic) testing is recommended. This testing looks for non-inherited gene mutations and other features of the cancer.

In people without an inherited *RET* mutation (or if this is unknown), testing the tumor for somatic (acquired) *RET* mutations is recommended.

The cancer should also be tested for tumor mutational burden-high (TMB-H), mismatch repair deficiency (dMMR), and microsatellite instability-high (MSI-H).

Treatment

Surgery is the preferred treatment for medullary thyroid cancer that returns to the neck area.

If the cancer can't be removed using surgery and is causing symptoms or getting worse, targeted therapy is often a treatment option. At this time, preferred targeted therapies include:

- Vandetanib (Caprelsa)
- Cabozantinib (Cabometyx)
- Selpercatinib (Retevmo) (for *RET* mutation-positive cancers)
- Pralsetinib (Gavreto) (for *RET* mutation-positive cancers)

The immunotherapy drug pembrolizumab (Keytruda) may be an option for TMB-H or dMMR/MSI-H tumors.

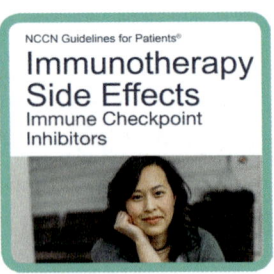

Immunotherapy side effects

Immune checkpoint inhibitors have unique side effects. Unlike other cancer treatments, the side effects of immunotherapy occur because the immune system is attacking healthy cells in the body.

Learning to recognize possible side effects can help you notice reactions early and report them to your care team.

More information on the side effects of immune checkpoint inhibitors is available at NCCN.org/patientguidelines and on the NCCN Patient Guides for Cancer app.

If treatment with surgery or systemic therapy isn't possible, external beam radiation therapy (EBRT) may be used instead.

Taking a watch-and-wait approach by monitoring the cancer can also be an appropriate option for some recurrent medullary thyroid cancers.

Metastatic cancer

Treatment of metastatic medullary thyroid cancer depends in part on whether the cancer is causing symptoms. If the cancer is stable and isn't causing symptoms, treatment may not be needed. Surgery, ablation, or other techniques to remove or destroy the metastases will be considered.

If the cancer progresses (gets worse) and begins causing symptoms, systemic therapy is often a treatment option. The same targeted therapies listed above are also preferred for metastatic disease. If the preferred therapies are not available or effective, other small-molecule kinase inhibitors may be considered. Chemotherapy that includes the drug dacarbazine (DTIC) may also be an option.

Radiation therapy may be used to help with symptoms, or as an ablative treatment in some cases. Surgery, ablation, or other techniques may be used to treat metastases in order to relieve symptoms.

If the cancer has spread to bone, intravenous bisphosphonates or denosumab are recommended. These are bone-strengthening medications that can help relieve symptoms and slow damage caused by bone metastases.

Joining a clinical trial is strongly encouraged for everyone with metastatic thyroid cancer. Ask your treatment team if there is an open clinical trial you might be eligible for.

Supportive care

Supportive care plays an essential role in the care of people with metastatic thyroid cancer. In addition to providing relief from symptoms caused by cancer and its treatment, supportive care can provide emotional, spiritual, and social support.

5 Medullary thyroid cancer » Key points

Key points

- Medullary thyroid cancer starts in the C cells of the thyroid. The C cells make a hormone called calcitonin.

- About 1 in 4 medullary thyroid cancers is inherited. Inherited medullary thyroid cancer is known as multiple endocrine neoplasia type 2 (MEN2). It is caused by mutations in the *RET* gene.

- Everyone diagnosed with medullary thyroid cancer using needle biopsy should be tested for *RET* mutations and offered genetic counseling. All medullary thyroid cancers are treated with total thyroidectomy.

- Blood tests to measure carcinoembryonic antigen (CEA) and calcitonin are recommended to monitor for the return of medullary thyroid cancer.

- Surgery is the preferred treatment for cancer that returns to the neck. Other options may include radiation therapy, monitoring (no treatment), and targeted therapy.

- Surgery, radiation therapy, or other techniques may be used to remove or destroy metastases and relieve symptoms.

- Supportive care can help relieve symptoms caused by medullary thyroid cancer and its treatment.

We want your feedback!

Our goal is to provide helpful and easy-to-understand information on cancer.

Take our survey to let us know what we got right and what we could do better.

NCCN.org/patients/feedback

6
Anaplastic thyroid cancer

42 Testing and staging

46 Non-metastatic ATC

47 Metastatic ATC

49 Important conversations

49 Monitoring and management

50 Key points

6 Anaplastic thyroid cancer » Testing and staging

Anaplastic carcinoma is the least common and most aggressive type of thyroid cancer. About half of people with this type have (or had) a more common type of thyroid cancer. Anaplastic thyroid cancer generally cannot be cured. Supportive care is essential throughout the treatment process.

Testing and staging

If a needle biopsy diagnoses anaplastic thyroid carcinoma (ATC), more testing is needed to confirm the diagnosis and learn the extent of the cancer. Testing typically includes blood tests and imaging procedures to see inside the head, neck, chest, abdomen, pelvis, voice box (larynx), and airway (trachea).

Biomarker testing

Testing the tumor for specific features, called biomarkers, is recommended for all anaplastic thyroid cancers. Testing helps determine whether you are eligible for treatment with targeted therapy or immunotherapy. Testing should include the biomarkers listed below.

- *BRAF* gene mutations
- *NTRK* gene fusions
- *ALK* gene fusions
- *RET* gene fusions
- DNA mismatch repair deficiency (dMMR)
- Microsatellite instability (MSI)
- Tumor mutational burden (TMB)

Staging

The results of imaging are used to determine the spread of cancer in the body, also known as the cancer stage.

All anaplastic thyroid cancers are stage IV (4). The letters A, B, and C are used to describe how far the cancer has spread at the time it is found.

Stages 4A and 4B are non-metastatic. If the cancer is only in the thyroid, it is stage 4A. If the cancer has grown into the neck or spread to nearby lymph nodes, it is stage 4B.

Stage 4C is metastatic disease. The cancer has spread to areas of the body far from the thyroid, such as the lungs or bone.

6 Anaplastic thyroid cancer » Testing and staging

Stage 4A

In stage 4A anaplastic thyroid cancer, the cancer has not grown or spread beyond the thyroid. The tumor may be small or large.

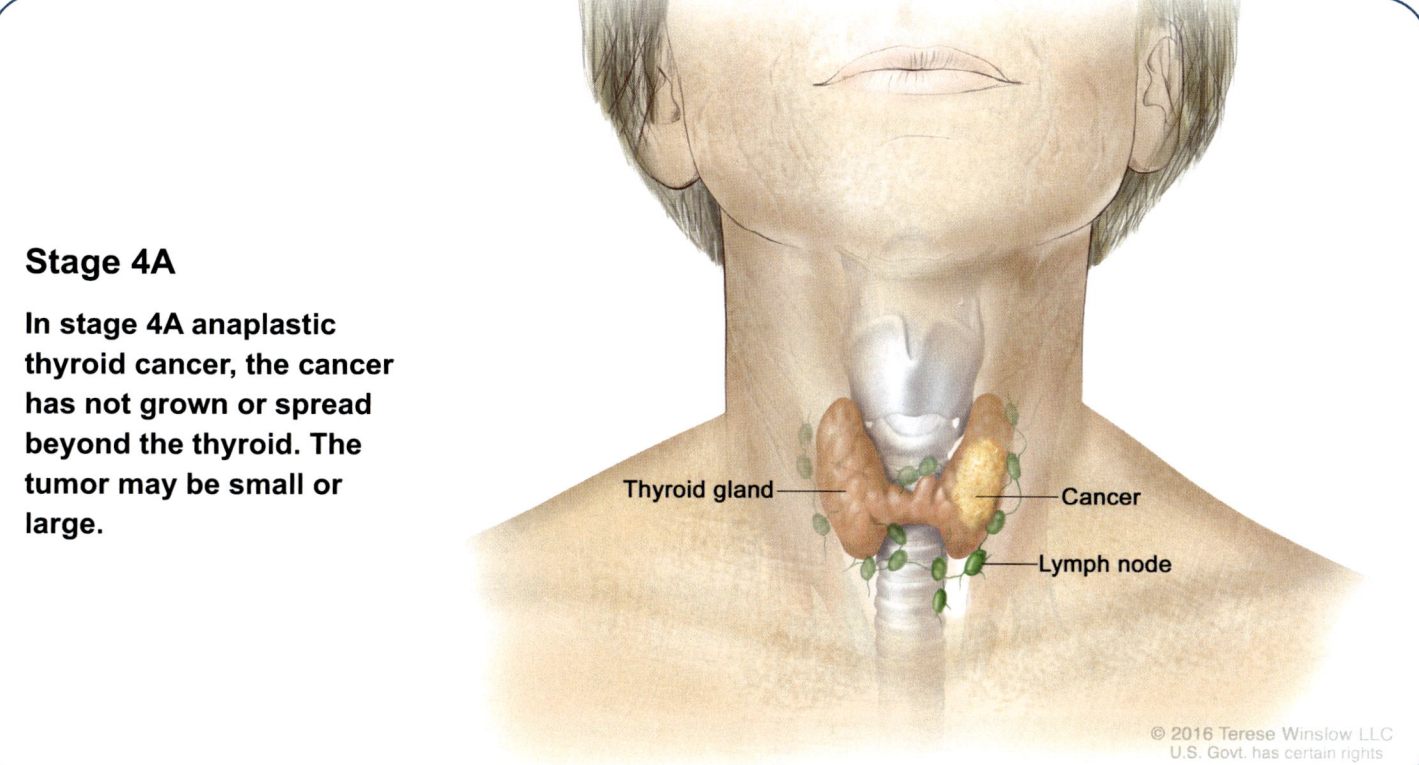

Stage 4B

In stage 4B anaplastic thyroid cancer, the cancer may have spread only to nearby lymph nodes, as shown here.

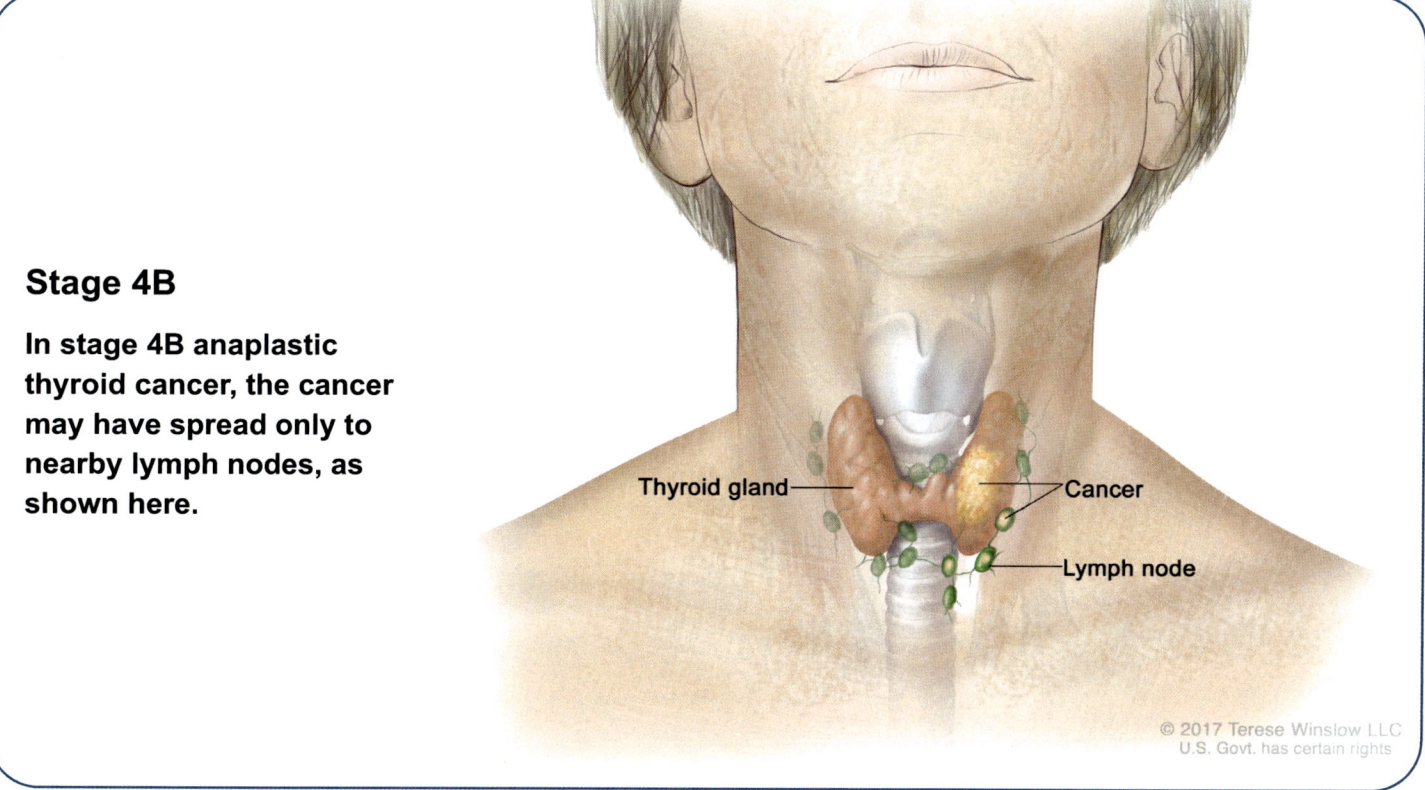

6 Anaplastic thyroid cancer » Testing and staging

Stage 4B (cont.)

Stage 4B also describes ATC that has grown into neck muscles next to the thyroid (top right) or grown extensively into th (bottom right).

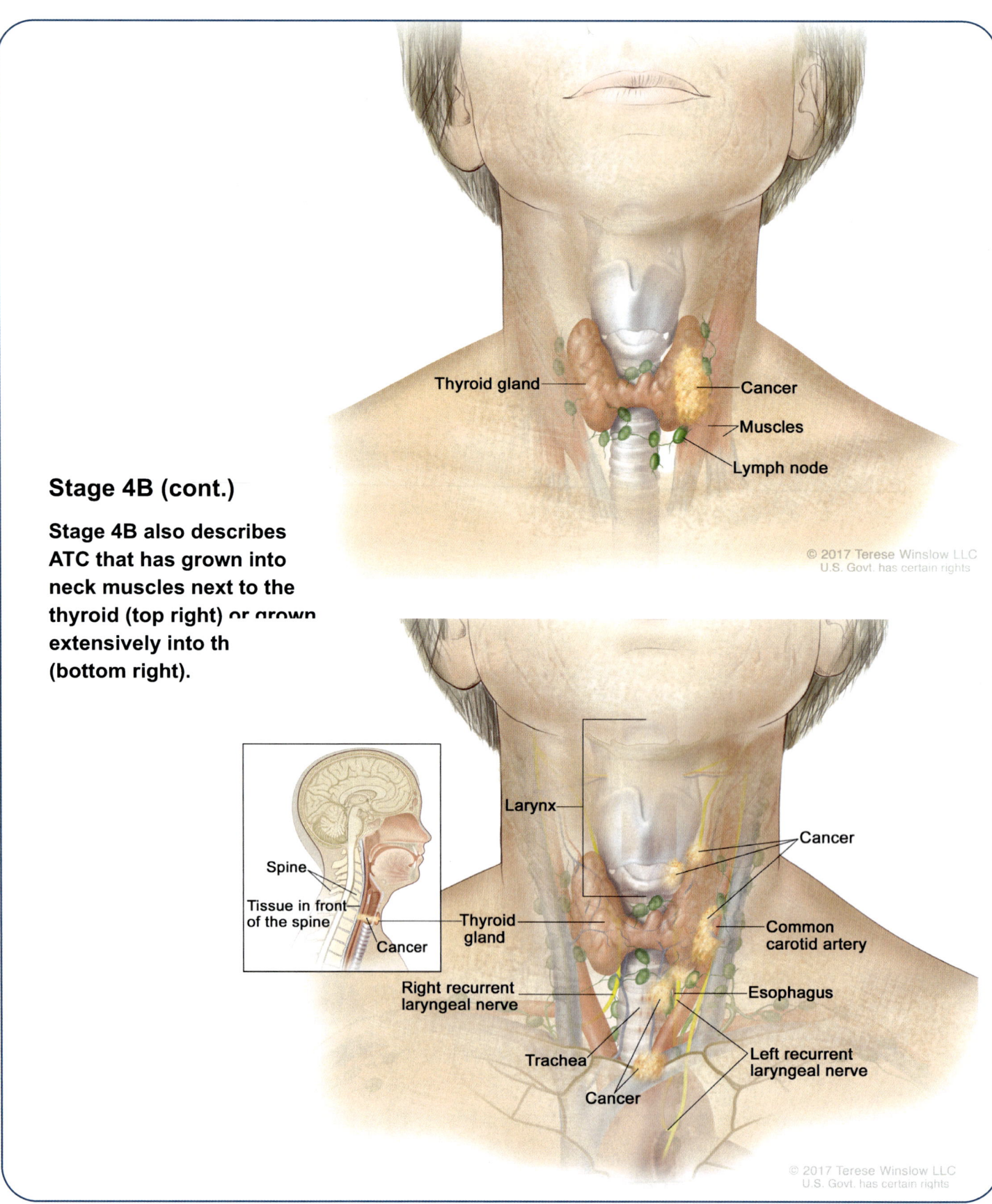

Stage 4C

Stage 4C is metastatic disease. The cancer has spread to areas of the body far from the thyroid.

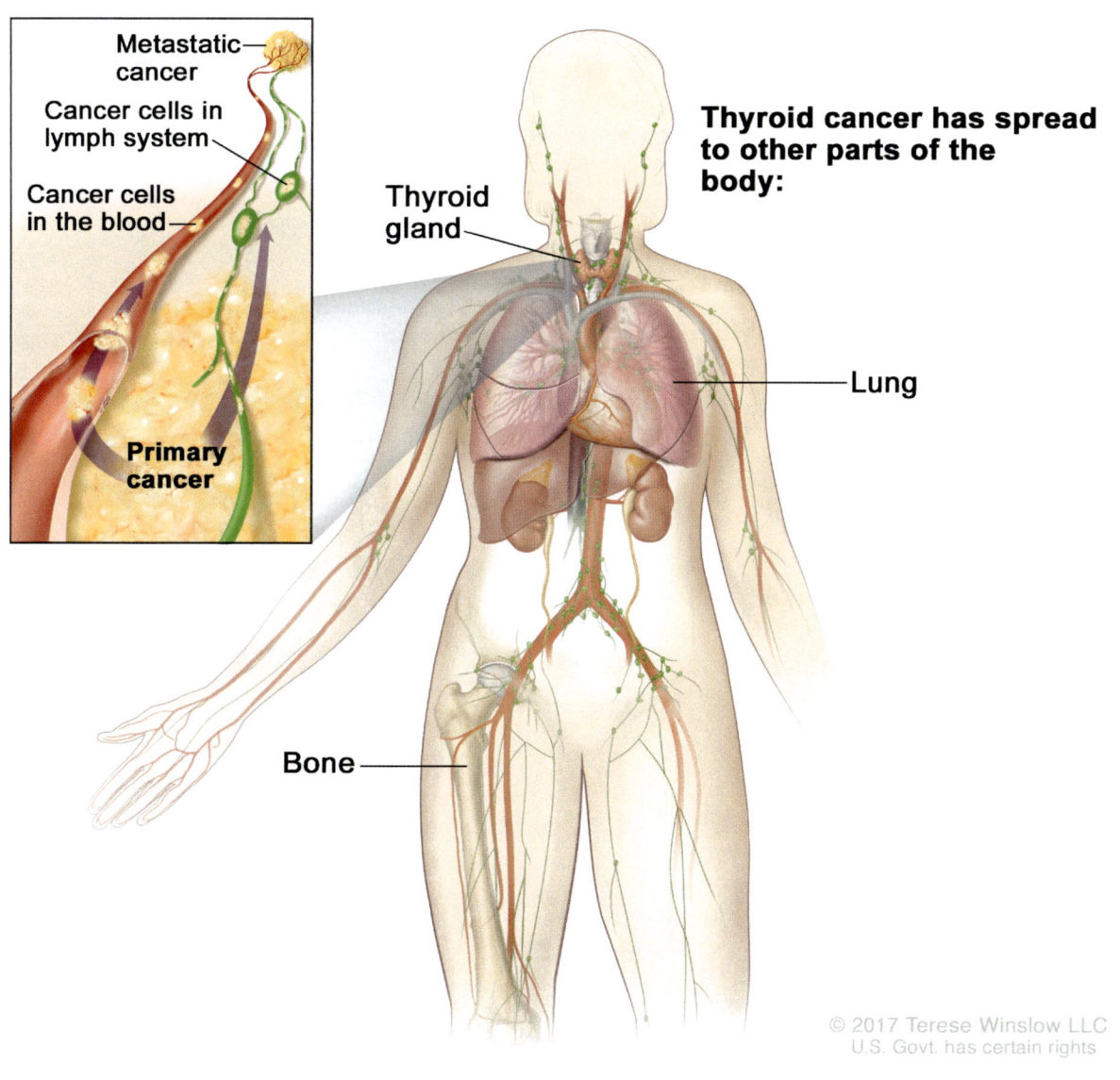

Non-metastatic ATC

Non-metastatic anaplastic thyroid cancer includes stages 4A and 4B. Treatment depends on whether the tumor can safely be removed using surgery. If it can, the entire thyroid is removed (total thyroidectomy). Nearby lymph nodes known or suspected to have cancer are also removed.

For cancers with a mutation in the *BRAF* V600E gene, targeted therapy may be given first to shrink the cancer before surgery. The recommended regimen is dabrafenib (Tafinlar) + trametinib (Mekinist).

If surgery successfully removes all of the cancer, or if only tiny amounts remain, external beam radiation therapy (EBRT) is next. EBRT kills microscopic leftover cancer cells in and around the cancer site.

Your doctor may recommend chemotherapy in addition to EBRT. When given with radiation, some chemotherapy medicines make it easier for radiation to kill cancer cells. This is called radiosensitizing chemotherapy. Treatment with both EBRT and chemotherapy during the same time period is known as chemoradiation.

A 2- to 3-week recovery period is recommended after surgery, before EBRT (and possibly also chemotherapy) is started.

If surgery isn't an option

If the cancer can't be safely removed using surgery, EBRT is recommended. Chemotherapy may be given in addition to radiation therapy.

The cancer may be borderline resectable. This means that surgery isn't an option right away due to the size and/or location of the tumor, but it may become possible. In this case, if the cancer has any of the biomarkers listed below, your doctor may recommend treatment with targeted therapy.

Recommended targeted therapies are listed below by biomarker:

- *BRAF* V600E mutation: Dabrafenib (Tafinlar) + trametinib (Mekinist)
- *RET* fusion-positive tumors: Selpercatinib (Retevmo) or pralsetinib (Gavreto)
- *NTRK* gene fusion-positive tumors: Larotrectinib (Vitrakvi) or entrectinib (Rozlytrek)

After treatment with either radiation therapy or targeted therapy, surgery may become an option. This will depend on the size of the tumor after treatment and other factors.

Metastatic ATC

If anaplastic thyroid cancer spreads to distant areas of the body, there may be more than one approach to treatment. Some people choose to treat the cancer aggressively. Others choose to maximize their quality of life. Talk to your care team about the approach that aligns with your health and personal preferences.

Anaplastic thyroid cancer grows quickly and can become quite large. Over time, the tumor may block the airway or cause other airway-related problems. Hoarseness, noisy breathing (stridor), and shortness of breath are possible signs of a blocked airway.

Whether you choose to treat the cancer aggressively or to maximize quality of life, your doctor may suggest tracheostomy. Tracheostomy is surgery to create an opening (called a stoma) in the windpipe. This surgery is typically done in an operating room under general anesthesia. An incision called a tracheotomy is made into the trachea (windpipe). A curved tube is placed into the newly created opening (the tracheostomy). The tracheostomy tube provides an airway used for breathing.

The decision to have a tracheostomy, and when, can be a difficult one for those with ATC and their caregivers. Your care team can provide information on the benefits and risks of

Guide 2
Systemic therapy for stage 4C (metastatic) anaplastic thyroid cancer

Preferred options for cancers with certain biomarkers	• ***BRAF* V600E-mutated cancers:** Dabrafenib (Tafinlar) + trametinib (Mekinist) • ***NTRK* gene fusion-positive cancers:** Larotrectinib (Vitrakvi) or entrectinib (Rozlytrek) • ***RET* fusion-positive cancers:** Selpercatinib (Retevmo) or pralsetinib (Gavreto)
Recommended options for cancers without above biomarkers	• Chemotherapy with paclitaxel, alone or with carboplatin • Chemotherapy with doxorubicin, alone or with docetaxel
May be recommended in certain situations	• Chemotherapy with doxorubicin and cisplatin • TMB-H cancers: Pembrolizumab (Keytruda) • Pembrolizumab + lenvatinib • Nivolumab (Opdivo)

6 Anaplastic thyroid cancer » Metastatic ATC

tracheostomy for you, taking into consideration your cancer and goals.

Option: Aggressive treatment

If you and your care team decide on this option, all of the following treatments may be used together to fight the cancer:

- Total thyroidectomy and lymph node dissection
- Radiation therapy
- Systemic therapy with or without radiation therapy **(see Guide 2)**

Joining a clinical trial may be another option. Participation in clinical trials is strongly encouraged for all patients with metastatic anaplastic thyroid cancer. Ask your treatment team if there are any open trials that you may be eligible for.

Option: Maximize quality of life

Aggressive treatment isn't an option for everyone with metastatic anaplastic thyroid cancer. It may not be recommended for health reasons, or it may not align with your preferences. Everyone's cancer and priorities are different. For some, living as comfortably as possible for as long as possible is preferred to undergoing treatments that may change your quality of life.

In this approach, the thyroid is not removed. Surgery, radiation therapy, or both are used to control cancer growth throughout the body. Removing or destroying areas of cancer directly can help relieve symptoms caused by cancer in the neck or distant areas.

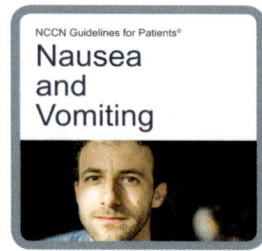

Chemotherapy side effects

Systemic therapy kills both cancer cells and healthy cells. The damage to healthy cells can cause hair loss, cracked skin, mouth sores, and other side effects.

Managing side effects is a shared effort between you and your care team. It is important to speak up about bothersome side effects, such as nausea and vomiting. Ask about your options for managing or relieving the effects of treatment.

More information on supportive care is available at NCCN.org/patientguidelines and on the NCCN Patient Guides for Cancer app.

If anaplastic thyroid cancer has spread to bones, denosumab (Prolia) or medications called bisphosphonates may be given to help strengthen your bones, slow bone damage, and relieve symptoms caused by the tumors.

Supportive care plays an essential role in the care of patients with anaplastic thyroid cancer. See *Chapter 7: Survivorship* for more information on the range of care that is available and important for cancer survivors.

Important conversations

Important, often difficult, discussions are needed after a diagnosis of anaplastic thyroid cancer. These discussions can help with making decisions about treatment and other care.

Prognosis

Prognosis refers to the expected outcome or course of an individual cancer. The prognosis for most anaplastic thyroid cancers is poor, meaning that good outcomes are unlikely.

Discussing prognosis is an important part of care planning for anaplastic thyroid cancer. Your prognosis can affect the type and number of treatments that you may be willing, or able, to receive.

Weigh treatment options

Consider and discuss the goals of treatment with your care team. Care to improve quality of life may be more helpful than cancer treatment. Talk to your doctor about your treatment options. For example, controlling the tumor growth may be preferred to aggressive treatment. Participation in clinical trials is strongly recommended for all patients with anaplastic thyroid cancer. Talk to your treatment team about clinical trials you may be eligible for.

Palliative care

Supportive care is available for everyone with anaplastic thyroid cancer. Supportive care can provide relief from symptoms as well as emotional, social, and spiritual support. Your doctor may suggest hospice care during this time.

Hospice care can help with the physical and emotional needs of anaplastic thyroid cancer. See *NCCN Guidelines for Patients: Distress During Cancer Care*, available at NCCN.org/patientguidelines and on the NCCN Patient Guides for Cancer app.

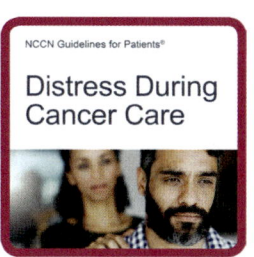

Monitoring and management

Imaging procedures (CT or MRI) of the brain, neck, chest, abdomen, and pelvis are needed on a regular basis for metastatic anaplastic thyroid cancer. There isn't a one-size-fits-all schedule for these scans. Talk to your treatment team about how often you need imaging. A combined PET/CT scan may be ordered 3 to 6 months after treatment of metastatic disease to determine the extent of the cancer.

If surveillance testing continues to find no evidence of disease (NED), monitoring will continue. Surgery, radiation therapy, or both are used to control cancer growth throughout the body. If the cancer returns or gets worse (progresses), trying a different systemic therapy may be an option. Joining a clinical trial is strongly encouraged if one is available to you.

Survivorship

In addition to surveillance testing, a range of other care is important for cancer survivors. See *Chapter 7: Survivorship* for more information.

6 Anaplastic thyroid cancer » Key points

Key points

- Anaplastic thyroid carcinoma (ATC) is the least common and most aggressive type of thyroid cancer.

- All anaplastic thyroid cancers are stage 4. The letters A, B, and C are used to describe how far the cancer has spread at the time it is found. Stages 4A and 4B are non-metastatic. Stage 4C is metastatic.

- If surgery is possible, non-metastatic ATC is treated with total thyroidectomy and lymph node dissection. Radiation therapy, and sometimes also chemotherapy, is used to kill cancer cells remaining after surgery.

- If surgery isn't an option, treatment with radiation therapy (and possibly chemotherapy) is recommended. If the cancer has biomarkers, treatment with targeted therapy may be an option instead of radiation therapy.

- For borderline resectable cancers, shrinking the tumor with targeted therapy or possibly immunotherapy may be an option. If treatment with radiation therapy or targeted therapy works well, surgery may become possible.

- Treatment of metastatic anaplastic thyroid cancer may focus on maximizing quality of life rather than treating the cancer. Aggressive therapy includes total thyroidectomy, radiation therapy, and systemic therapy.

- Supportive care is essential for everyone with anaplastic thyroid cancer. It can help relieve the side effects of cancer and its treatment. It can also provide mental, social, and spiritual care and support.

Supportive care is available for everyone with cancer. It isn't meant to treat the cancer, but rather to help with symptoms and make you more comfortable.

7
Survivorship

52 Paying for care

52 Your primary care provider

53 Healthy habits

54 More information

54 Key points

7 Survivorship

Survivorship focuses on the physical, emotional, and financial issues faced by cancer survivors. Managing the long-term side effects of cancer and its treatment, staying connected with your primary care provider, and living a healthy lifestyle are important parts of survivorship.

Thyroid cancer survivors may experience long-term health effects of cancer and its treatment. Such side effects can include:

- Osteoporosis
- High blood pressure
- Heart rhythm disorders
- Heart valve disease

These effects are different for everyone and depend in part on the treatment(s) received. Surgery, radiation therapy, radioactive iodine (RAI) therapy, and hormone replacement therapy all have unique potential side effects.

Paying for care

Cancer survivors face a unique financial burden. Paying for doctor visits, tests, and treatments can become unmanageable, especially for those with little or no health insurance. You may also have costs not directly related to treatment, such as travel expenses and the cost of childcare or missed work.

The term financial toxicity is used to describe the problems patients face related to the cost of medical care. Financial toxicity can affect your quality of life and access to needed health care. If you need help paying for your cancer care, financial assistance may be available. Talk with a patient navigator, your treatment team's social worker, and your hospital's financial services department.

Your primary care provider

After finishing cancer treatment, your oncologist and primary care provider should work together to make sure you get needed follow-up care. Ask your oncologist for a written survivorship care plan. Ideally, the plan will include:

- A summary of your cancer treatment history
- A description of possible late- and long-term side effects
- Recommendations for monitoring for the return of cancer
- Clear roles and responsibilities for your providers
- Recommendations on your overall health and well-being

7 Survivorship » Healthy habits

Healthy habits

It is important to keep up with other aspects of your health after cancer treatment. Steps you can take to help prevent other health problems and to improve your quality of life are described next.

Cancer screening

Get screened for other types of cancer, such as breast, colorectal, and skin cancer. Your primary care provider can tell you what cancer screening tests you should have based on your age and risk level.

Other health care

Get other recommended health care for your age, such as blood pressure screening, hepatitis C screening, and immunizations (like the flu shot).

Diet and exercise

Try to exercise for at least 150 minutes per week. This will help you stay at a healthy body weight.

Alcohol may increase the risk of certain cancers. Drink little to no alcohol. Eat a diet rich in plant-based foods.

Quit smoking

If you smoke or vape, tell your care team. They can help you find a way to quit that works for you.

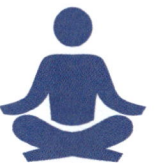

Complementary and alternative therapies

Complementary and alternative therapies may help with side effects and improve comfort and well-being during and after cancer treatment. Some of these practices and products include:

Acupuncture

Dietary supplements

Eastern medicine

Medical marijuana

Herbal teas and preparations

Homeopathy

Hypnosis

Meditation

Reiki

Yoga

Massage therapy

If you have questions or are curious about complementary therapies, talk to your treatment team. Many cancer centers have integrative oncology programs. Integrative oncology is an approach to cancer care that combines conventional (standard) cancer treatment with complementary and alternative therapies.

More information

For more information on cancer survivorship, the following are available at NCCN.org/patientguidelines and on the NCCN Patient Guides for Cancer app:

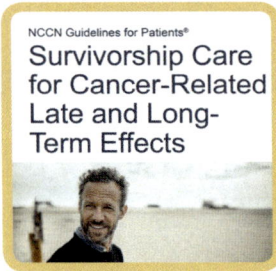
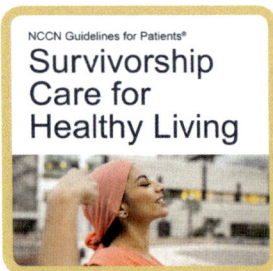

> *Survivorship Care for Healthy Living*
> *Survivorship Care for Cancer-Related Late and Long-Term Effects*

These resources address many topics relevant to cancer survivors, including:

> Anxiety, depression, and distress
> Fatigue
> Pain
> Sexual health
> Sleep problems
> Healthy lifestyles
> Immunizations
> Work, insurance, and disability concerns

Key points

> Survivorship focuses on the physical, emotional, and financial issues unique to cancer survivors.

> Your oncologist and primary care doctor should work together to make sure you get the follow-up care you need.

> A survivorship care plan is helpful in transitioning your care to your primary care doctor.

> Healthy habits, including exercising and eating nutritious foods, play an important role in helping to prevent other diseases and second cancers.

8
Making treatment decisions

56 It's your choice

56 Questions to ask

62 Resources

8 Making treatment decisions » It's your choice

It's important to be comfortable with the cancer treatment you choose. This choice starts with having an open and honest conversation with your doctor.

It's your choice

In shared decision-making, you and your doctors share information, discuss the options, and agree on a treatment plan. It starts with an open and honest conversation between you and your doctor.

Treatment decisions are very personal. What is important to you may not be important to someone else. Some things that may play a role in your decision-making:

> What you want and how that might differ from what others want

> Your religious and spiritual beliefs

> Your feelings about certain treatments like surgery or chemotherapy

> Your feelings about pain or side effects such as nausea and vomiting

> Cost of treatment, travel to treatment centers, and time away from work

> Quality of life and length of life

> How active you are and the activities that are important to you

Think about what you want from treatment. Discuss openly the risks and benefits of specific treatments and procedures. Weigh options and share concerns with your doctor.

If you take the time to build a relationship with your doctor, it will help you feel supported when considering options and making treatment decisions.

Second opinion

It is normal to want to start treatment as soon as possible. While cancer should not be ignored, there is time to have another doctor review your test results and suggest a treatment plan. This is called getting a second opinion, and it's a normal part of cancer care. Even doctors get second opinions!

Things you can do to prepare:

> Check with your insurance company about its rules on second opinions. There may be out-of-pocket costs to see doctors who are not part of your insurance plan.

> Make plans to have copies of all your records sent to the doctor you will see for your second opinion.

Support groups

Many people diagnosed with cancer find support groups to be helpful. Support groups often include people at different stages of treatment. If your hospital or community doesn't have support groups for people with cancer, check out the websites listed in this book.

Questions to ask

Possible questions to ask your doctors are listed on the following pages. Feel free to use these or come up with your own.

8 Making treatment decisions » Questions to ask

Questions about testing

1. What tests will I have for thyroid cancer?

2. Where and when will the tests take place?

3. How long will they take?

4. What are the risks?

5. How do I prepare for testing?

6. How soon will I know the results and who will explain them to me?

7. Have any cancer cells spread to other parts of my body?

8. Can you tell me about the symptoms of thyroid cancer?

9. What will happen if the thyroid nodule isn't cancer?

8 Making treatment decisions » Questions to ask

Questions about treatment

1. What are my treatment options? Which do you recommend?

2. Does this hospital or center offer the best treatment for me?

3. Will my age, general health, and other factors affect my treatment choices?

4. How much time do I have to think about my options? Is there time to get a second opinion?

5. What can I do to prepare for treatment?

6. How long will I be in the hospital after surgery? How soon can I return to my normal activities?

7. What symptoms should I look out for during treatment?

8. How much will the treatment cost? How can I find out how much my insurance company will cover?

9. How likely is it that I'll be cancer-free after treatment?

10. What is the chance that the cancer will come back?

8 Making treatment decisions » Questions to ask

Questions about side effects

1. What are the side effects of surgery?

2. What are the side effects of radioactive iodine (RAI) therapy?

3. What are the side effects of external beam radiation therapy (EBRT)?

4. What are the side effects of systemic therapy?

5. When can side effects start? How long will they last?

6. When should I contact the care team about my side effects?

7. Are there any medications that can prevent or relieve these side effects?

8. Are there any long-term effects of this treatment?

8 Making treatment decisions » Questions to ask

Questions about clinical trials

1. Is there a clinical trial I can join?

2. What is the purpose of the study?

3. How many people will be in the clinical trial?

4. What are the tests and treatments for this study (including placebos)? How often will they take place?

5. Has the treatment been used before? Has it been used for other types of cancers?

6. What side effects can I expect from the treatment? Can the side effects be controlled?

7. How long will I be in the clinical trial?

8. How will you know the treatment is working?

9. Will I be able to get other treatment if this treatment doesn't work?

10. Who will help me understand the costs of the clinical trial?

8 Making treatment decisions » Questions to ask

Questions about resources and support

1. Who can I talk to about help with housing, food, and other basic needs?

2. What help is available for transportation, childcare, and home care?

3. How much will I have to pay for treatment?

4. What help is available to pay for medicines and treatment?

5. What other services are available to me and my caregivers?

6. How can I connect with others and build a support system?

7. How can I find in-person or online support?

8. Who can help me with my concerns about missing work or school?

9. Who can I talk to if I don't feel safe at home, at work, or in my neighborhood?

10. How can I get help to stop smoking or vaping?

8 Making treatment decisions » Resources

Resources

AnCan
Ancan.org

Bone Marrow & Cancer Foundation
Bonemarrow.org

CancerCare
Cancercare.org

Cancer Hope Network
Cancerhopenetwork.org

Imerman Angels
Imermanangels.org

National Coalition for Cancer Survivorship
canceradvocacy.org

THANC Foundation
Thancfoundation.org

ThyCa: Thyroid Cancer Survivors' Association, Inc.
thyca.org

Triage Cancer
Triagecancer.org

U.S. National Library of Medicine Clinical Trials Database
clinicaltrials.gov

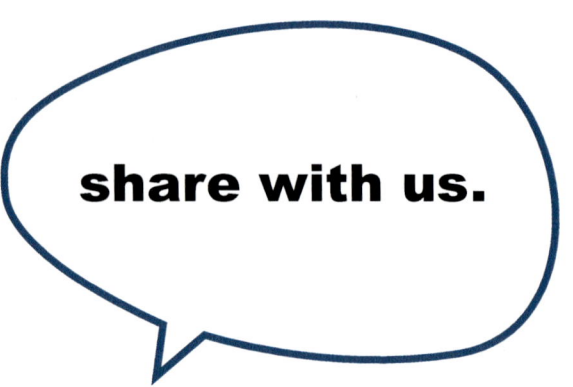

Take our survey and help make the NCCN Guidelines for Patients better for everyone!

NCCN.org/patients/comments

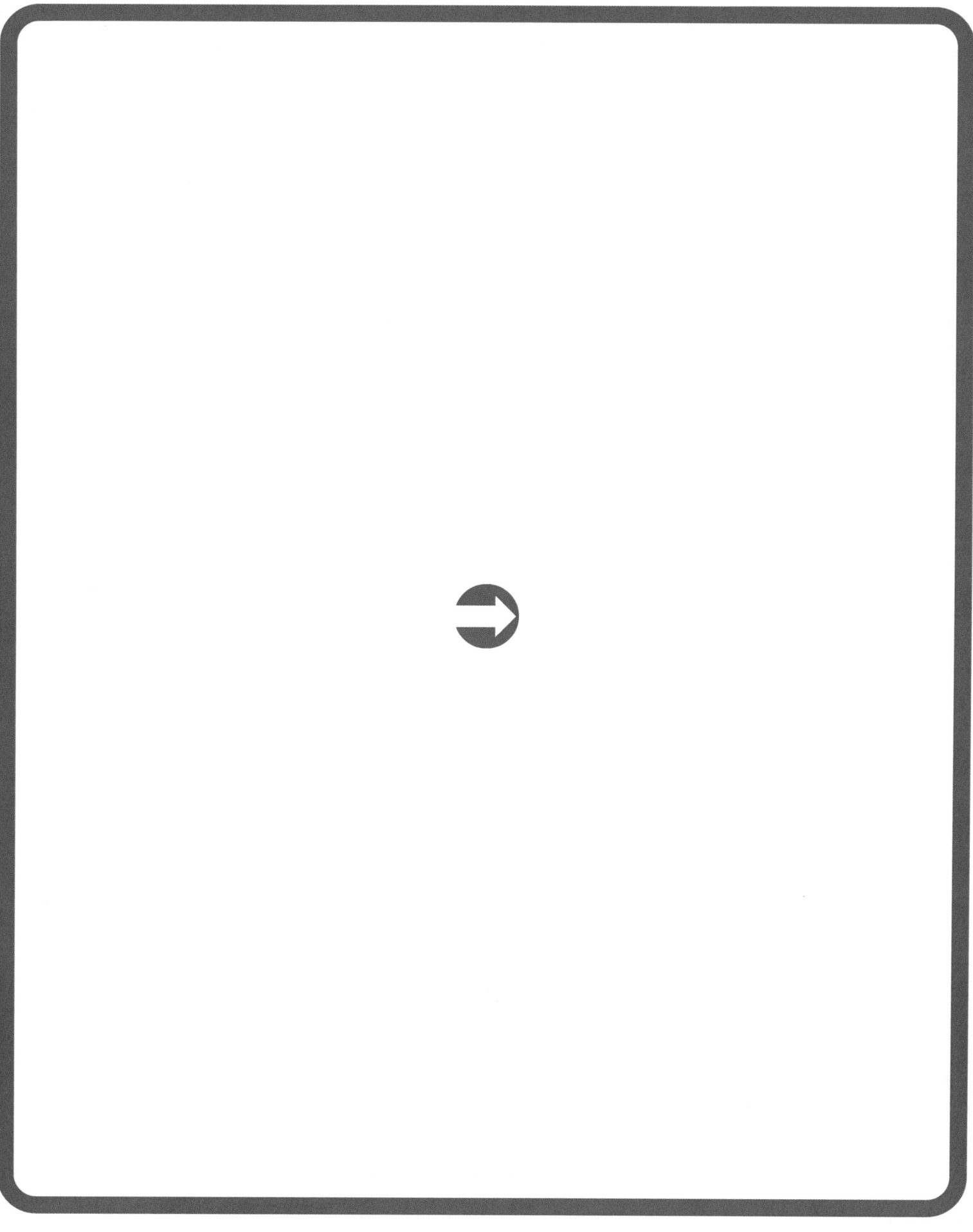

Words to know

anaplastic thyroid cancer
A rare and aggressive type of thyroid cancer. Anaplastic cells look very different from normal thyroid cells. Also called anaplastic thyroid carcinoma (ATC).

biomarkers
A feature of a cancer that may be targetable. Many are mutations (changes) in the DNA of the cancer cells.

biopsy
Removal of small amounts of tissue or fluid to be tested for disease.

C cells
Cells in the thyroid that make calcitonin. These cells are also called parafollicular cells.

calcitonin
A hormone made by the C cells of the thyroid gland. It helps control the calcium level in the blood.

chemotherapy
Drugs that work throughout the body to kill cancer cells.

clinical trial
Research on an investigational test or treatment to assess its safety or how well it works.

computed tomography (CT)
A test that uses x-rays to view body parts.

contrast
A substance put into your body to make clearer pictures during imaging tests.

follicular thyroid cancer
The second most common type of thyroid cancer. Starts in follicular cells and invades blood vessels in and around the thyroid. Also called follicular thyroid carcinoma (FTC).

oncocytic thyroid cancer
An uncommon and often more aggressive type of differentiated thyroid cancer. Used to be called Hürthle cell carcinoma (HCC).

magnetic resonance imaging (MRI)
A test that uses radio waves and powerful magnets to make pictures of the insides of the body.

medullary thyroid cancer
A type of thyroid cancer that starts in the C cells that make calcitonin. About 1 out of 4 medullary thyroid cancers is caused by inherited mutations of the *RET* gene. Also called medullary thyroid carcinoma (MTC).

metastasis
The spread of cancer cells from the first tumor to another body part.

neck dissection
Removal of the lymph nodes and other tissue in the neck area.

nodule
A small mass of abnormal tissue.

noninvasive follicular thyroid neoplasm with papillary-like nuclear features (NIFTP)
A low-risk, noninvasive thyroid tumor. Formerly known as encapsulated follicular variant of papillary thyroid cancer.

Words to know

observation
A period of scheduled follow-up testing to watch for signs of cancer spread (metastasis) or return (recurrence).

papillary thyroid cancer
The most common type of thyroid cancer. Starts in follicular cells. Also called papillary thyroid carcinoma (PTC).

parathyroid gland
One of 4 small glands near the thyroid that make parathyroid hormone.

pathologist
An expert in examining cells and tissues to diagnose disease.

pathology report
A document with information about cells and tissues removed from the body and examined with a microscope for disease.

pituitary gland
A gland found near the base of the brain. It makes hormones that control how other glands in the body work or make hormones.

positron emission tomography (PET)
A test that uses radioactive material to see the shape and function of body parts.

PTEN hamartoma tumor syndrome (PHTS)
An inherited syndrome that can cause follicular thyroid cancer and other cancers and health problems. Also called Cowden syndrome.

supportive care
Care given to improve the quality of life of patients who have a serious or life-threatening disease. Also called palliative care.

stereotactic radiosurgery (SRS)
A non-surgical and highly precise type of radiation therapy that can be used to treat small brain or spine tumors.

stereotactic body radiation therapy (SBRT)
A special ablative radiation technique that delivers high doses of radiation to precise areas to kill cancer cells.

thyroid
A gland located beneath the larynx (voice box) that makes thyroid hormone and calcitonin. The thyroid gland helps regulate growth and metabolism.

Thyrogen
A form of thyroid-stimulating hormone (TSH) made in a lab. It is used to test for remaining or recurring cancer cells in patients who have been treated for thyroid cancer. Also called thyrotropin alfa.

thyroid hormone
Refers to the 2 main hormones made by the thyroid: thyroxine (T4) and triiodothyronine (T3). The thyroid uses a mineral from your diet called iodine to produce these hormones.

tumor
An abnormal mass of cells.

whole brain radiation therapy (WBRT)
A type of external radiation therapy used to treat cancer in the brain.

NCCN Contributors

This patient guide is based on the NCCN Clinical Practice Guidelines in Oncology (NCCN Guidelines®) for Thyroid Carcinoma, Version 3.2024. It was adapted, reviewed, and published with help from the following people:

Dorothy A. Shead, MS
Senior Director
Patient Information Operations

Erin Vidic, MA
Senior Medical Writer, Patient Information

Susan Kidney
Senior Graphic Design Specialist

The NCCN Guidelines® for Thyroid Carcinoma, Version 3.2024 were developed by the following NCCN Panel Members:

Robert I. Haddad, MD/Chair
Dana-Farber/Brigham and Women's Cancer Center | Mass General Cancer Center

Lindsay Bischoff, MD/Vice-Chair
Vanderbilt-Ingram Cancer Center

Sarimar Agosto Salgado, MD
Moffitt Cancer Center

Megan Applewhite, MD
The UChicago Medicine Comprehensive Cancer Center

Victor Bernet, MD
Mayo Clinic Comprehensive Cancer Center

Erik Blomain, MD, PhD
Stanford Cancer Institute

Naifa Lamki Busaidy, MD
The University of Texas MD Anderson Cancer Center

Michael Campbell, MD
UC Davis Comprehensive Cancer Center

Paxton Dickson, MD
The University of Tennessee Health Science Center

Quan-Yang Duh, MD
UCSF Helen Diller Family Comprehensive Cancer Center

Hormoz Ehya, MD
Fox Chase Cancer Center

Whitney S. Goldner, MD
Fred & Pamela Buffett Cancer Center

Erin Grady, MD
Stanford Cancer Institute

Theresa Guo, MD
UC San Diego Moores Cancer Center

Megan Haymart, MD
University of Michigan Rogel Cancer Center

Shelby Holt, MD
UT Southwestern Simmons Comprehensive Cancer Center

Jason P. Hunt, MD
Huntsman Cancer Institute at the University of Utah

Fouad Kandeel, MD, PhD
City of Hope National Medical Center

Dominick M. Lamonica, MD
Roswell Park Comprehensive Cancer Center

Jochen Lorch, MD
Robert H. Lurie Comprehensive Cancer Center of Northwestern University

Susan J. Mandel, MD, MPH
Abramson Cancer Center at the University of Pennsylvania

Stephanie Markovina, MD, PhD
Siteman Cancer Center at Barnes-Jewish Hospital and Washington University School of Medicine

*Lisle Nabell, MD, PhD
O'Neal Comprehensive Cancer Center at UAB

Christopher D. Raeburn, MD
University of Colorado Cancer Center

Rod Rezaee, MD
Case Comprehensive Cancer Center/ University Hospitals Seidman Cancer Center and Cleveland Clinic Taussig Cancer Institute

John A. Ridge, MD, PhD
Fox Chase Cancer Center

Hadley Ritter, MD
Indiana University Melvin and Bren Simon Comprehensive Cancer Center

*Mara Y. Roth, MD
Fred Hutchinson Cancer Center

Randall P. Scheri, MD
Duke Cancer Institute

Jatin P. Shah, MD, PhD
Memorial Sloan Kettering Cancer Center

*Jennifer A. Sipos, MD
The Ohio State University Comprehensive Cancer Center - James Cancer Hospital and Solove Research Institute

Rebecca Sippel, MD
University of Wisconsin Carbone Cancer Center

Cord Sturgeon, MD
Robert H. Lurie Comprehensive Cancer Center of Northwestern University

Lori J. Wirth, MD
Mass General Cancer Center

Richard J. Wong, MD
Memorial Sloan Kettering Cancer Center

*Francis Worden, MD
University of Michigan Rogel Cancer Center

Michael W. Yeh, MD
UCLA Jonsson Comprehensive Cancer Center

NCCN Staff

Susan Darlow, PhD
Manager, Guidelines Information Standardization

Carly J. Cassara, MSc
Guidelines Layout Specialist

* Reviewed this patient guide. For disclosures, visit NCCN.org/disclosures.

NCCN Cancer Centers

Abramson Cancer Center
at the University of Pennsylvania
Philadelphia, Pennsylvania
800.789.7366 • pennmedicine.org/cancer

Case Comprehensive Cancer Center/
University Hospitals Seidman Cancer Center and
Cleveland Clinic Taussig Cancer Institute
Cleveland, Ohio
UH Seidman Cancer Center
800.641.2422 • uhhospitals.org/services/cancer-services
CC Taussig Cancer Institute
866.223.8100 • my.clevelandclinic.org/departments/cancer
Case CCC
216.844.8797 • case.edu/cancer

City of Hope National Medical Center
Duarte, California
800.826.4673 • cityofhope.org

Dana-Farber/Brigham and Women's Cancer Center |
Mass General Cancer Center
Boston, Massachusetts
877.442.3324 • youhaveus.org
617.726.5130 • massgeneral.org/cancer-center

Duke Cancer Institute
Durham, North Carolina
888.275.3853 • dukecancerinstitute.org

Fox Chase Cancer Center
Philadelphia, Pennsylvania
888.369.2427 • foxchase.org

Fred & Pamela Buffett Cancer Center
Omaha, Nebraska
402.559.5600 • unmc.edu/cancercenter

Fred Hutchinson Cancer Center
Seattle, Washington
206.667.5000 • fredhutch.org

Huntsman Cancer Institute at the University of Utah
Salt Lake City, Utah
800.824.2073 • healthcare.utah.edu/huntsmancancerinstitute

Indiana University Melvin and Bren Simon
Comprehensive Cancer Center
Indianapolis, Indiana
888.600.4822 • www.cancer.iu.edu

Mayo Clinic Comprehensive Cancer Center
Phoenix/Scottsdale, Arizona
Jacksonville, Florida
Rochester, Minnesota
480.301.8000 • Arizona
904.953.0853 • Florida
507.538.3270 • Minnesota
mayoclinic.org/cancercenter

Memorial Sloan Kettering Cancer Center
New York, New York
800.525.2225 • mskcc.org

Moffitt Cancer Center
Tampa, Florida
888.663.3488 • moffitt.org

O'Neal Comprehensive Cancer Center at UAB
Birmingham, Alabama
800.822.0933 • uab.edu/onealcancercenter

Robert H. Lurie Comprehensive Cancer Center
of Northwestern University
Chicago, Illinois
866.587.4322 • cancer.northwestern.edu

Roswell Park Comprehensive Cancer Center
Buffalo, New York
877.275.7724 • roswellpark.org

Siteman Cancer Center at Barnes-Jewish Hospital
and Washington University School of Medicine
St. Louis, Missouri
800.600.3606 • siteman.wustl.edu

St. Jude Children's Research Hospital/
The University of Tennessee Health Science Center
Memphis, Tennessee
866.278.5833 • stjude.org
901.448.5500 • uthsc.edu

Stanford Cancer Institute
Stanford, California
877.668.7535 • cancer.stanford.edu

The Ohio State University Comprehensive Cancer Center -
James Cancer Hospital and Solove Research Institute
Columbus, Ohio
800.293.5066 • cancer.osu.edu

The Sidney Kimmel Comprehensive
Cancer Center at Johns Hopkins
Baltimore, Maryland
410.955.8964
www.hopkinskimmelcancercenter.org

The UChicago Medicine Comprehensive Cancer Center
Chicago, Illinois
773.702.1000 • uchicagomedicine.org/cancer

The University of Texas MD Anderson Cancer Center
Houston, Texas
844.269.5922 • mdanderson.org

UC Davis Comprehensive Cancer Center
Sacramento, California
916.734.5959 • 800.770.9261
health.ucdavis.edu/cancer

NCCN Cancer Centers

UC San Diego Moores Cancer Center
La Jolla, California
858.822.6100 • cancer.ucsd.edu

UCLA Jonsson Comprehensive Cancer Center
Los Angeles, California
310.825.5268 • uclahealth.org/cancer

UCSF Helen Diller Family Comprehensive Cancer Center
San Francisco, California
800.689.8273 • cancer.ucsf.edu

University of Colorado Cancer Center
Aurora, Colorado
720.848.0300 • coloradocancercenter.org

University of Michigan Rogel Cancer Center
Ann Arbor, Michigan
800.865.1125 • rogelcancercenter.org

University of Wisconsin Carbone Cancer Center
Madison, Wisconsin
608.265.1700 • uwhealth.org/cancer

UT Southwestern Simmons Comprehensive Cancer Center
Dallas, Texas
214.648.3111 • utsouthwestern.edu/simmons

Vanderbilt-Ingram Cancer Center
Nashville, Tennessee
877.936.8422 • vicc.org

Yale Cancer Center/Smilow Cancer Hospital
New Haven, Connecticut
855.4.SMILOW • yalecancercenter.org

Notes

Index

ablation 31, 39

active surveillance 13, 23

ALK gene fusion 30, 42

BRAF gene mutation 30–31, 42, 46–47

calcitonin 34–37

clinical trial 19–20, 60

Cowden syndrome 7

genetic counseling 34–35

levothyroxine 13–14, 23–24, 26–28, 31, 36

immunotherapy 18, 30–31, 38, 42

mismatch repair (MMR) 30, 38, 42

noninvasive follicular thyroid neoplasm with papillary-like nuclear features (NIFTP) 25

NTRK gene fusion 30–31, 42, 46–47

osteoporosis 52

pheochromocytoma 34, 37

RET mutation 34, 36, 38

stereotactic radiosurgery (SRS) 32

Thyrogen 16

tracheostomy 47–48

tumor mutational burden (TMB) 30–31, 38, 42, 46–47

vitamin D 14

whole brain radiation therapy (WBRT) 32

Made in the USA
Las Vegas, NV
04 October 2025

29068388R00043